EVELINE SMITH

I0146030

Intermittent Fasting For Women Over 50

Join The Excitement And Achieve A Youthful, Slim Frame - Discover Do's And Do-Not's For A Smooth Journey To Weight Loss!

Table of Contents

Chapter 1. A Brief Introduction To Intermittent Fasting

You may have heard about Intermittent Fasting from your friends, or maybe some random talk show mentioned it as some fat loss miracle. You've overheard some women at the gym bringing it up during their chat about carb-cycling and protein shakes. But what is it? The name says it all. Intermittent-periods; fasting - being without food. What's so special about periods without food? Every time I say the word fasting to my relatives, they get this big fearful look on their faces as if I am starving myself and could die at any moment! Fortunately, you won't be starving yourself. It's not one of those fasts that last 30 days and have you drinking lemonade and spices.

In essence, Intermittent Fasting is a strategy to make dieting easier. How does it do that? Well, let's define dieting. I'll bring this up again later, but, to lose weight, you have to eat less than you are eating right now. That's a challenge for people because people's usual method is to start giving up the things they love. They start eating tiny salads, give up their cheeseburgers, and it starts to become painful. So what happens? They fail. We have all done it. You want to be healthy, but your day is already full of stress, and food is your outlet (well, it's mine anyway!); it helps you wind down. It is where the magic of intermittent Fasting can save the day. Don't eat after dinner until the following day at lunch, shifting you're eating into a smaller window of time. What does this do? It lets you eat big, satisfying meals but is ultimately less food than you would typically eat. And boom! Dieting is not so hard after all. Now, I know I'm leaving out lots of details. You might be shouting at this book right now thinking, No, breakfast is important! Fasting will put my body in starvation mode!

Before understanding what intermittent Fasting amounts to, you need to know that Intermittent Fasting is not a diet fad. Instead, it is a dieting pattern. To put it clearly, Intermittent Fasting is making a well-thought-out decision to skip or avoid individual meals and fasting for certain periods. It means a specific period or "window" of a certain number of hours where you are allowed to eat. Simultaneously, there is a larger fasting window of more hours where you need to eat nothing. So, you skip meals and eat smaller portions, and you will start shedding those pounds in no time at all. Well, that is only half the truth. Yes, by cutting down a meal, you reduce the average calories that you consume for a week – even if you eat more than usual during your feeding window. However, you need to keep in mind that all the calories in the world are not equal! Consuming calories from carbs have a different effect on the body than consuming calories from fats!

Another factor that plays a significant role in the timing of the meals that you consume.

Chapter 2. How Does Intermittent Fasting Work?

While following Intermittent Fasting, your body follows a different operational mode while the body is in a fasting state to that which is used in the feasting state. But how does this work? Whenever you consume a meal, it takes your body a couple of hours to process the food you have finished and burn whatever it can from processed food. Due to this, your body has a tremendous amount of energy to burn, fueling the body instead of using fat. It happens when you consume sugar or carbs, as these are the primary sources of glucose. As the glucose molecule is the easiest to synthesize for energy, the body burns the glucose first before moving on to more challenging burn energy stores.

While your body is in a fasting state, your body does not have readily available energy from the food you have consumed. So, in such a case, your body is forced to break down the stored fat in itself to keep the body fueled, and the bodily functions are going. It is because, over the hours of Fasting, the body has already used up all the glucose and glycogen derived from the food that you have consumed while you were permitted to eat. So, the body has no other option but to use the energy that has been stored in the form of fats in the body.

But why does this method work so efficiently? Well, the body reacts to the food we consume by producing insulin. When your body is sensitive to insulin, there is a more efficient use of the energy consumed. It not only helps with losing weight but also helps in the creation of muscle mass. While you are fasting, your insulin sensitivity is at its peak. When you are asleep, your body uses the glycogen stored in the liver and muscles to fuel the body. The glycogen is exhausted throughout the night. Your body expects you to eat food first thing in the morning to replenish your glycogen levels again. By skipping breakfast, you do not provide the body with glycogen, thus increasing insulin sensitivity. So, when you finally eat, everything you eat is used more efficiently because the glycogen you consume is used to create muscle mass and is burned to provide your body with energy – thus leaving very little for your body to store as fat! When you compare this to standard, non-fasting days, you will understand the actual impact intermittent fasting has on the body!

When you aren't fasting, your body's insulin sensitivity is at a reasonable level. So, when you consume foods rich in sugar and carbs, your body's glycogen levels will max out. There will be a high level of glucose in the bloodstream that is enough to keep your body energized. So, all the extra glycogen is converted to fat and is stored in multiple places in your body. But, when you fast, the glycogen reserves in the body go down, forcing your body to release growth hormone. It, combined with increased insulin sensitivity and a decreased insulin production level, helps you gain muscle mass while losing some fat from your body. To put it very clearly, intermittent Fasting helps regulate your bodily functions. It uses the food you consume more efficiently and burns fats to be used as fuel when you are not continually consuming calories. Due to various physiological reasons, when done correctly, Fasting helps build muscle and promote weight loss.

Body fat is the body's system of saving energy (calories). When we don't consume something, the body alters many things to make the preserved extra power available. Intermittent Fasting formulates instinctive sense. The food we eat is digested by catalysts in our gut and ends up as molecules in our blood system. Starches, especially sugars and refined grains (white flours and rice), are immediately converted into sugar (glucose), which our cells use for the essentials. If our cells don't use glucose totally, it is stored in our fat cells. Glucose enters our cells with insulin (a hormone made in the pancreas). Insulin conveys glucose into the fat cells and keeps it there. If we eat less, our insulin levels will go down, and our fat cells would then be able to discharge their preserved sugar to be utilized as vitality. The whole thought of it is to permit the insulin levels to go down to burn kept fat.

This fact has to do with alterations in nervous system function and the most significant variation in most crucial hormones.

"One of the main keys to comprehend fasting, and to comprehend any diet, is comprehending the function insulin plays," Dr. Hutchins says. Insulin, the hormone that controls blood sugar, is made in the pancreas and discharged into the bloodstream in reaction to carbohydrate consumption. Once released, insulin causes the body to preserve energy as fat. "Insulin formulates fat, so the more insulin made, the more fat you preserve," he says. When you are not expanding in irregular Fasting, give the body time to diminish insulin levels, which inverses the fat-protecting framework. "When insulin levels fall, the system goes in reverse, and you decline fat."

Two different hormones, ghrelin, and leptin are additionally grinding away. Ghrelin is the hunger hormone. "A few pieces of information propose that intermittent fasting can diminish ghrelin," Dr. Hutchins says. "There's also a little information that says there's an enhancement in leptin, which is the satiety hormone. That is the one that acquaints us with the sensation "I'm full". With extra leptin and less ghrelin, individuals will feel full quicker and hungry less regularly, which could mean fewer calories devoured and, therefore, weight reduction. Discontinuous Fasting or Intermittent Fasting (IF) may appear to be new, yet it's taken from an old idea. Our predecessors had everyday times of Fasting, mainly when nourishment was rare or inaccessible. Nowadays, in any case, nourishment sources are ample. Presently, Intermittent Fasting has become a psychological practice alongside a method for diminishing irritation and conceivably decreasing your hazard for specific conditions, such as diabetes. Individuals even report that their thinking becomes clearer, and their cognitive processes have improved because of Intermittent Fasting.

Even though it might decrease insulin, irregular Fasting can bring adrenaline and cortisol up in specific individuals. These two hormones play a fundamental role in numerous necessary capabilities, similar to digestion, muscle aggravation, and memory. After some time, in specific people, up-graded cortisol can prompt cortisol dysregulation, or, a few sources state, adrenal fatigue. Your body formulates cortisol from cholesterol. If that level remains high for a long time, it will, in the end, the body will use progesterone, a sex hormone, to keep itself going. Inevitably, elevated cortisol can cause reactions like decreased sex hormones (progesterone), muscle weakness, cerebral pains, weight addition, and sleep deprivation. It can likewise influence the measure of thyroid-stimulating hormone (TSH) that you make, which can additionally slow your digestion. A few types of discontinuous or intermittent Fasting may provoke extreme calorie limitation if you're not cautious. Having an over the top calorie deficiency for a long time can adversely affect estrogen and luteinizing hormone in certain ladies, which may cause unpredictable or missing cycles.

Body fat is the body's system of saving energy (calories). When we don't consume something, the body alters many things to make the preserved extra power available. Using intermittent Fasting makes intuitive sense.

Chapter 3. Effect Of Intermittent Fasting On Physiology

There is some proof that irregular fasting may not help some women as much as it does for men. One study demonstrated that glucose control deteriorated in women following three weeks of discontinuous fasting, and this same finding was not true in the male subjects.

Likewise, numerous accounts of women who have encountered changes to their feminine cycles following initiation of discontinuous fasting. Such changes can happen because female bodies are very sensitive to calorie limitation. At the point when calorie intake is low —, for example, when fasting for a long time or too frequently — the nerve center of the brain is influenced.

It can disturb the discharge of gonadotropin-delivering chemicals (GnRH). This chemical helps discharge two conceptive chemicals: luteinizing hormone (LH) and follicle stimulating hormone (FSH). At the point when these chemicals can't communicate with the ovaries, you risk irregular periods, feelings of lethargy, and in addition to other impacts on your overall wellbeing, you will weaken bone structures. Even though there are no comparable human investigations, tests in rodents have demonstrated that 3–6 months of substitute day fasting caused a decrease in ovary size and irregular regenerative cycles in female rodents.

Hence, women need to consider a different way to deal with discontinuous fasting. For example, women will find more success with more limited fasting periods and fewer fasting days than their male counterparts.

Synopsis

Irregular fasting may not be as advantageous for women in comparison to men. To diminish any unfavorable impacts, women should adopt a gentle strategy to fasting: using strategies such as more limited diets and fewer fasting days.

Medical advantages of Intermittent Fasting for Women

Irregular fasting benefits your waistline as well as lowering your chances of acquiring various chronic health conditions.

Heart Health

Coronary illness is the primary source of death around the world.

Hypertension, high LDL cholesterol, and increased fats in your blood are the main risk factors that need to be addressed for improving coronary health.

One investigation in 16 overweight people demonstrated irregular fasting brought down circulatory stresses by 6% in only two months.

Likewise, a similar report found that irregular fasting brought down LDL cholesterol by 25% and fatty substances by 32%.

Nonetheless, the proof for the connection between irregular fasting and improved LDL cholesterol and fatty oil levels isn't predictable.

An examination in 40 average weight individuals found that a month of discontinuous fasting during the Islamic occasion of Ramadan didn't bring about a decrease in LDL cholesterol or fatty substances.

More high quality examinations using robust techniques are required before specialists can thoroughly comprehend the impacts of discontinuous fasting on the wellbeing of the heart.

Diabetes

Irregular fasting may likewise successfully contribute to a reduction in risk of developing diabetes. Like constant calorie limitation, intermittent fasting seems to reduce a portion of the risk factors for diabetes. It does so fundamentally by bringing down insulin levels and decreasing insulin resistance.

In a randomized, controlled investigation of more than 100 overweight women, a half year of irregular fasting diminished insulin levels by 29% and insulin resistance by 19%. Glucose levels were maintained. Furthermore, 8–12 weeks of discontinuous fasting appeared to bring down insulin levels by 20–31% and glucose levels by 3–6% in people with pre-diabetes.

In this condition, glucose levels are elevated, however not sufficiently high to diagnosed as diabetes.

Be that as it may, discontinuous fasting may not be as helpful for women in comparison to men for lowering glucose. A little report found that glucose control deteriorated for women following 22 days of substitute day fasting, while there was no antagonistic impact on glucose control for men.

Regardless of this result, the decrease in insulin and insulin resistance would, in any case, probably lessen the danger of diabetes, especially for people with pre-diabetes.

Weight reduction

Discontinuous fasting can be a straightforward and successful approach to get in shape when used appropriately, as daily transient diets can assist you with burning-through fewer calories and shedding pounds.

Various investigations propose that irregular fasting is as compelling as regular calorie-limited eating regimens for immediate weight reduction. A 2018 audit of studies in overweight grown-ups discovered intermittent fasting prompted an average weight reduction of 15 lbs (6.8 kg) over three years.

Another audit indicated discontinuous fasting decreased body weight by 3–8% in overweight or stout adults over a period of 3–24 weeks. The survey found that members decreased their abdominal girth by 3–7% over a similar period. It ought to be noted that the long term impacts of irregular fasting on weight reduction for women remains to be seen.

For the time being, discontinuous fasting appears to help in weight reduction. Notwithstanding, the amount you lose will probably rely upon the number of calories you burn-through during non-fasting periods and how long you commit to lifestyle.

It May Help You Eat Less

Changing to discontinuous fasting may generally assist you with eating habits. One investigation found that youngsters ate 650 fewer calories each day when their food intake was limited to a four-hour window.

Another investigation in 24 dependable people examined the impacts of a long, 36-hour fast on dietary patterns. Notwithstanding burning-through additional calories on the post-fast day, members dropped their complete calorie balance by 1,900 calories, which is quite a considerable decrease.

Other Health Benefits

Various human and animal studies recommend that discontinuous fasting may likewise yield other medical advantages.

• Reduced inflammation: Some examinations show that irregular fasting can decrease key markers of irritation. Constant inflammation can prompt weight gain and contribute to several medical conditions.

• Improved mental focus: One investigation found that two months of irregular fasting diminished despondency and overeating practices while improving self-perception in over weight adults.

• Increased life span: Intermittent fasting has appeared to expand life expectancy in rodents and mice by 33–83%. The impacts on the life span in people are yet to be resolved.

• Preserve bulk: Intermittent fasting has all the more compelling earmarks of holding muscle mass when contrasted with long term calorie restriction. Higher muscle mass encourages your body to consume more calories, even at rest.

In particular, the medical advantages of irregular fasting for women should be more broadly examined in large human studies before more conclusive findings are claimed.

Outline

Discontinuous fasting may assist women with getting slimmer and diminish their risk of coronary illness and diabetes. In any case, further human investigations are expected to affirm these discoveries.

Best Types of Intermittent Fasting for Women

When it comes to dieting, there is no one-size-fits-all approach. This truism also applies to intermittent fasting. Generally speaking, women should take a more relaxed approach to fasting than men. That approach may include shorter fasting periods, fewer fasting days, and consuming a smaller number of calories on the fasting days.

Here are some of the best types of intermittent fasting for women:

- Crescendo Method: Fasting 12–16 hours two to three days a week. Fasting days should be nonconsecutive and spaced evenly across the week (Monday, Wednesday, and Friday).
- Eat-stop-eat (also called the 24-hour protocol): A 24-hour full fast once or twice a week (maximum of two times a week for women). Start with 14–16 hour fasts and gradually build up.
- The 5:2 Diet (also called "The Fast Diet"): Restrict calories to 25% of your usual intake (about 500 calories) for two days a week and eat "normally" the other five days. Allow one day between fasting days.
- Modified Alternate-Day Fasting: Fasting every other day but eating "normally" on non-fasting days. You are allowed to consume 20–25% of your usual calorie intake (about 500 calories) on a fasting day.
- The 16/8 Method (also called the "Leangains method"): Fasting for 16 hours a day and eating all of your calories within an eight-hour window. Women are advised to start with 14-hour fasts and eventually build up to 16 hours.

Whichever you choose, it is still essential to eat well during the non-fasting periods. Suppose you eat a large amount of unhealthy, calorie-dense foods during the non-fasting periods. In that case, you may not experience the same weight loss and health benefits.

The best approach that you can tolerate and sustain in the long-term should not result in any negative health consequences.

Rundown

There are numerous ways for women to do discontinuous fasting. The best techniques probably incorporate the 5:2 eating routine, adjusted substitute day fasting, and the crescendo strategy.

The beginning is necessary.

Odds are you've just done numerous irregular diets previously. Numerous individuals intuitively eat like this, skipping morning or night suppers. The most straightforward approach to begin is to pick one of the intermittent fasting strategies above and give it a go.

In any case, you don't have to follow an organized arrangement initially.

An option is to fast at whatever point it suits you—skipping suppers every once in a while when you don't feel hungry or don't have the opportunity to cook can work for specific individuals. It doesn't make a difference which sort of fast you pick. The main thing is to discover a technique that works out best for you and your way of life.

Synopsis

The easy method to begin is to pick one of the strategies noted and give it a go. Stop immediately if you do happen experience any negative side-effects.

Wellbeing and Side Effects

Altered adaptations of irregular fasting have all the signs of being safe and effective for most women.

That being said, a few investigations have revealed some adverse results, including hunger, mood swings, loss of focus, diminished energy, headaches, and bad breath on fasting days.

Likewise, a few reports of women indicating that their menstrual cycle stopped following a discontinuous fasting diet.

It would help if you talked with your Medical Doctor before attempting discontinuous fasting on the off chance you have a health condition that is worsened by fasting.

Clinical discussion is critical for women who:

• Have a background marked by dietary issues.

• Have diabetes or routinely experience low glucose levels.

• Are underweight, malnourished, or have nutritional deficiencies.

• Are pregnant, breastfeeding, or attempting to become pregnant?

• Have fertility issues or a history of amenorrhea (missed periods).

Discontinuous fasting seems to have a decent security profile. However, on the off chance that you experience any issues —, for example, losing your monthly cycle — do stop the practice right away.

Synopsis

Discontinuous fasting may cause hunger, low energy levels, migraines, and bad breath. Women who are pregnant, trying to conceive or have a background marked by dietary issues should look for clinical confirmation before beginning an irregular fasting routine.

The Bottom Line

Discontinuous fasting is a dietary example that includes ordinary, transient diets. The best kinds for ladies incorporate every day 14–16 hour diets, the 5:2 eating routine, or adjusted substitute day fasting.

While discontinuous fasting is beneficial for heart wellbeing, diabetes, and weight reduction, some evidence suggests it might negatively affect women who are attempting to get pregnant, and women with problems with their glucose levels. That being said, altered forms of discontinuous fasting seem appropriate for most women and might be a more appropriate choice than longer or stricter diets. If you are a woman hoping to get in shape or improve your wellbeing, discontinuous fasting is an option to consider in meeting your goals.

The advantages of discontinuous fasting

It shouldn't be assumed that discontinuous fasting doesn't have a useful role to play in weight loss and maintenance. Discontinuous fasting may work for specific individuals, Aronne adds, particularly if they would prefer not to be messing with calorie counting and food records. "It's not my best option for weight reduction," he says, "however I have discovered that in a select gathering of patients attempting to get in shape, having them eat all their food in eight hours works for them since it's simple and they don't need to consider everything: They take care of business."

For everybody, it is recommended, for the most part, to eat to augment your circadian rhythms — your body's internal clock that guides you to wake and rest — however much as could reasonably be expected, exhorts Michael Roizen, M.D., Chief Wellness Officer of the Cleveland Clinic and creator of What to Eat When. "Our bodies advance to be prepared for food during the day with the goal that we have a lot of energy for endurance," he says. Therefore, your body is generally touchy to the presence of insulin. This chemical moves glucose from your blood into cells for energy and capacity during the day and it is usually impervious to it around evening time. Overlooking these rhythms and eating at some unacceptable occasions — such as around late evening time — can raise glucose, a risk factor for type 2 diabetes, as per a study directed by specialists at Harvard University and Brigham Women's Hospital.

Adopt a strategy instead of making breakfast (or, if you can't stomach eating a great deal that early, lunch) the primary meal of the day, and make your supper a light one after the sun goes down. "This conveys a large number of similar advantages to those of irregular fasting since for the most part you're not eating inside a 12-hour window. However, it's a lot simpler," clarifies Roizen.

Chapter 4. How IF Affects Hormones, Serum Lipid Levels, Coagulation Status, and Plasma Homocysteine Levels.

Notably, nutritional habits, resting examples, and frequency of meals affect the maintenance of human wellbeing. In the Ramadan period that is a holy month, all Muslims abstain from drinking and eating during daylight hours. The little nourishment and drink ingestion for around 12h/day, typical of Ramadan, is a particular discontinuous fasting model. Numerous physiological and mental changes are most likely because of Ramadan's progressions in feeding and sleep schedules. Homocysteine is a blended amino acid, and acts as a go-between on the metabolic pathway between methionine and cysteine.

Some B nutrients are cofactors in the methionine catabolic pathway. And deficiencies in folic acid, vitamin B12, and pyridoxine have been related to somewhat raised homocysteine levels in large numbers of people. The capacity of plasma homocysteine levels in vascular infections and these mechanisms remain are a matter of study. Some investigations suggest that hyper-homocysteinemia may animate procoagulant factors or disable anticoagulant components in our circulating blood by influencing ordinary cell capacities. D dimer refers to a protein fragment of fibrin that can be detected in the blood following the breakdown of a blood clot (this breakdown is called fibrinolysis). Fibrin is a mesh that holds proteins together, and D dimer (the leftovers of this protein connection matrix) are measured through blood tests that help health teams detect thrombosis or the presence of blood clotting. Circulating levels of D dimer reflects the degree of fibrin turnover in the blood. Henceforth, plasma D dimer levels show fibrin age and fibrinolytic action in the body. It indicates that fibrin D dimer is related to the risk of future ischemic coronary illness in people with and without existing symptoms of vascular disorder.

Physiological changes in delayed irregular Fasting and the potential impacts of postponed or abbreviated occasions of rest on human digestion are not entrenched. The effects of IF and the adjustment in resting digestion on serum lipid levels, coagulation status, and plasma homocysteine levels have been explored. In an examination led by Fehime Benli Aksunga, long-enduring modifications in the circadian patterns of the eating and resting schedules were brought about by the different timing of digestion, and Ramadan fasting changes appeared to affect metabolic endocrine systems. In the current study, our subjects had similar working hours before and during Ramadan. As indicated by the survey, during Ramadan their bedtime was postponed on average by two hours.

There were two significant changes in their daily schedule: supper timing and bedtime. The absence of substantial bodyweight change demonstrates that nourishment consumption from dusk to dawn was sufficient to balance vitality. Then again, in the daylight hours, fasting subjects should undoubtedly be experiencing a lack of hydration. Yet, as confirmed from the body weight and the poll, there was no interminable dehydration during Ramadan among our subjects. Hydration levels appeared to be regulated as the 24-hour urinary volumes didn't change significantly. This finding is consistent with those in another ongoing investigation utilizing an isotopic tracer strategy, it has been demonstrated to save all-out body water content in Ramadan fasting. Late tests with people and animals with moderate hyper-homocysteinemia gave an understanding of the component underlying minor rises of homocysteine and vascular illness. These studies showed the likelihood that raised homocysteine is multifactorial, influencing both the vascular cell walls and blood coagulation framework.

A meta-analysis by the Homocysteine Studies Collaboration confirmed homocysteine is a risk factor for the first occasions of stroke and coronary heart disease (CHD). These outcomes show that homocysteine levels were decreased in the most recent seven-day stretch of Ramadan and returned nearly to the baseline levels 20 days after Ramadan. None of our subjects utilized any supplements. As per the poll, utilization of nourishment containing folic acid and other B nutrients didn't change significantly during the investigation.

Ramadan's adjustments in the sleep-wake cycle as well as rest and nourishment patterns may beneficially influence the bio-availabilities or redistribution of cofactors like B nutrients. In any case, systems that underlie homocysteine lessen in intermittent Fasting for 15 h/day for a month, as in the Ramadan fasting model, and thus must be additionally researched as some previous found slight hyper-homocysteinemia.

Under fasting conditions there is a minor impairment in the methylation pathway, even though the fasting conditions were distinctive in these investigations. In the present research, there was a significant reduction in D dimer levels in Fasting. It proposes that slightly raised D dimer levels reflect minor upgrades in blood coagulation, thrombin development, and a turnover of cross-connected intravascular fibrin, which is mostly intra-blood vessel. These increases might contribute to coronary heart disease (CHD) as past planned investigations recommend that CHD risk is roughly 70% more noteworthy in those with higher plasma D dimer levels. Aybak et al. showed that Ramadan fasting prompted a decrease in the platelet responses to various factors. A similar report had revealed an upgrade in draining and coagulation time (however, not significant). These outcomes are in concurrence with the current investigation.

What's more, plasma factor VII coagulant action (FVIIc) exhibits higher levels following a meal and stayed elevated for seven hours, particularly following high-fat meals. In Ramadan fasting, one feast is over-looked; consequently, you may not see a potential improvement in FVIIc movement after lunch. Moreover, the relationship between homocysteine and fibrin D dimer is under scrutiny in more recent studies. In a multivariate investigation, the association of homocysteine and D dimer is demonstrated to remain factually significant after modification for constant inflammation and fibrinogen. These outcomes are predictable with our examination. We demonstrated a significant decrease in D dimer levels, showing the decreased fibrin age in the body during intermittent Fasting. Also, homocysteine levels connect with D dimer levels. In combination with different up until now less reliable instruments, such as upgraded HDL levels, coagulation initiation might be negligible in drawn-out discontinuous Fasting.

Plasma fibrinogen and D dimer levels were not correlated in our study. Past investigations have announced significant connections between plasma D dimer and fibrinogen levels. This absence of connection has been accounted for by the decrease in quality of the relationship between high D dimer levels and CHD, showing that D dimer is a free risk factor for CHD. Then again, it estimated cuttable fibrinogen. Sweetnam et al. reported that a warm precipitation nephelometric measure of fibrinogen has a high exhibition in insignificant varieties and anticipates CHD. No different reports on plasma D dimer, fibrinogen, and homocysteine levels in Ramadan fasting are accessible as far as anyone is aware. A large portion of the past investigations on Ramadan fasting didn't utilize female subjects – in the present study both female and male subjects were included.

The prohibition of fasting in the menstrual time (5, 8, 2 day periods) is by all accounts without impact. The data from female subjects is comparable to that from participants. Studies have demonstrated that ten days were essential for the body to adjust metabolically to resting propensities in any event. Moreover, it shows that metabolic changes continue as before for ten days after Ramadan. In the present study, 5, 8, 2 day periods were conceivably insufficient for the metabolic change, which might explain fasting interference in the menstrual time, not influencing our data. In our investigation, the practically raised serum HDL levels. The HDL risk factor was altogether diminished in Ramadan and continued as before 20 days after Ramadan in both female and male subjects. The change in expending tendencies in Ramadan didn't influence different lipoproteins, TC, and TG levels. These outcomes are reliable with the study by Adlouni et al.. Still, in their studies, Maislos et al. reported that HDL levels came back to baseline levels a month after the end of Ramadan. Twenty days after Ramadan may not be sufficient for HDL to go back to pre-fasting levels, which is a bit of leeway on the risk of coronary heat disease.

HDL's role in lipid digestion is the take-up and transport of cholesterol from peripheral tissues to the liver through a framework known as reverse cholesterol transport, which functions as a cardio-protective instrument. Low HDL levels are related to an increased risk of CHD. The multivariate investigation suggests that the best free lipid indicator of CHD risk among populations is the TC/HDL ratio (HDL risk factor). And an increase of the HDL risk factor adds an overabundance of 68% to both the non-deadly and lethal CHD event. The investigation took non-fasting tests in the first part of the day in addition to the evening's fasting levels.

This point impedes the present research, as some analyzed parameters have circadian varieties. In any case, homocysteine, D dimer, PT, aPTT, BUN, creatinine, and all-out protein levels don't generally change in a day. Another constraint in this study is just a single estimation for the D dimer levels toward the end of the fasting time. It could have concluded a different arrangement of D dimer measures to prevent errors in accuracy. Nonetheless, our outcomes show that this applied no nutritional eating regimen routine and no decrease in caloric intake to the subjects. Intermittent Fasting prompted some valuable changes in serum

HDL and homocysteine levels of coagulation status. It might expect these progressions to exclude at any rate one meal when the body was exceptionally metabolically dynamic and simultaneously conceivably had a low blood consistency level. We reason that intermittent Fasting may beneficially affect hemostatic risk factors for cardiovascular disease.

Chapter 5. Effect Of IF In Insulin

Fasting is the most proficient and reliable system to decrease insulin levels. This fact was first noted decades ago and evidence is broadly acknowledged. It is very straightforward and self-evident. All eating raises insulin, so the best technique for diminishing insulin is to take a break from ingesting food. Blood glucose levels stay regulated as the body starts to switch over to consuming fat for energy. This impact is with fasting times as short as 24-36 hours. Longer-term fasts lessen insulin even more significantly. Moreover, as of late, substitute day-by-day fasting has been consider as a satisfactory method to decreasing insulin in the system. Regular fasting, reducing insulin levels, has likewise been revealed to fundamentally improve insulin efficiency. This method is the missing link in the weight reduction challenge. Most weight loss regimens suggest people significantly reduce the intake of foods that require high levels of insulin in order to be used by the body, or high insulin dependent foods, but these regimens don't address the issue of insulin resistance.

In these regimens weight is at first lost; however, insulin resistance keeps insulin levels and the body Set Weight high. Fasting is a useful technique for diminishing insulin resistance, and decreasing insulin causes the collection of an overabundance of salt and water preserved in the kidney. Atkins-style consumption of fewer calories regularly causes diuresis, the loss of water retention, prompting the dispute that a significant part of the underlying weight reduction is actually water and not fat. While diuresis is genuinely helpful in lessening swelling and feeling 'lighter' and some may likewise experience a marginally lower heart rate. Fasting additionally is found to have an early time of successful and quick weight reduction. For the initial five days, weight reduction a median level of 0.9 kg/day, far surpassing the method of simple caloric limitation. This result is likely because of the impact of diuresis, or reduction of salt and water shed in these early stages of the regimen.

Growth hormone

Growth hormone is known to improve the accessibility and utility of fats for fuel. It additionally assists with saving muscle mass and maintaining bone density. Growth hormone production lessens consistently with age. One of the most potent ways to increase hormone production is through fasting. Over a five-day fast, growth hormone production becomes many times higher. The net physiologic impact is to keep up muscle and bone tissue mass over the fasting time. It is precisely this development of a hormone flood that contributes to cell regeneration. Long haul investigations of intermittent fasting demonstrate that the fasting methodology is more significantly better at safeguarding lean mass rate when contrasted with regimens that only use calorie restriction.

Chapter 6. Change In Fat Tissue Morphology, Physiology And Distribution

Fat tissue in your body is fundamental to the maintenance of glucose and lipid balance. It also acts as a significant sink and capacity organ for FFA (Free Fatty Acids) and a wellspring of various adipocytes equipped for impacting entire body digestion. Factors influencing weight-related metabolic issues are multivariate and include a tendency for affected individuals to gain weight when under psychological stress; obese individuals store more fat; macrophage penetration brings about secondary inflammation and impairs the use of stored fat for energy; increasing insulin resistance as well as circulating lipids in the blood; and this continues to cause excess fat to be stored. These outcomes make for an ominous metabolic and hormonal milieu, which drives the work to improve of foundational insulin resistance and related metabolic disorders. A few investigations have indicated that rodents kept up on IER (Intermittent Energy Restriction) display diminished instinctive fat tissue and significant decreases in overweight cell size, and increased adipocyte separation inside subcutaneous and instinctive fat pads. However, adiponectin levels, which have antiatherogenic and insulin-sharpening properties, are generally diminished in corpulent conditions, but improved through IER. Considering one examination, these valuable changes in fat tissue physiology and morphology seem to be equivalent to CER (Continuous Energy Restriction), but what was one of a kind to IER is that it didn't require a general vitality shortage, which is maybe owing to the exchanging times of taking care of and fasting. One uncontrolled exchange day completed fasting discovered improved insulin-intervened lipolysis restraint in human subjects, reflecting improved insulin activity, after two weeks.

Notwithstanding decreases in absolute adiposity, IER weight reduction has detailed decreases in instinctive fat tissue, truncal adiposity, and gainful changes in circling adipocyte profiles. For instance, pro-atherogenic adipocytes, including leptin, are decreased, while adiponectin levels are enhanced. Among studies contrasting changes in fat tissue measures (complete, truncal, and midriff circumference) and circulating adipocytes among IER and CER, no steady comparison have been observed. Be that as it may, extra investigations utilizing vigorous appraisals of obesity are required.

Electrolytes

Worries about a lack of healthy sustenance in fasting are understandable, but not supported by evidence. Inadequate calories are not a significant stress since fat stores are adequate.

The primary concern is the development of a lack of micronutrients. However, even long term investigation of fasting have uncovered no proof of ailing health. Potassium levels may lessen somewhat, yet even two months of persistent fasting doesn't decrease levels below 3.0 mEq/L, even without the utilization of supplements. This length of fasting is far longer than, for the most part, suggested in intermittent fasting regimens. Magnesium, calcium, and phosphorus levels in fasting remain normal. Probably, due to the enormous reserves of these minerals in the bones. Ninety-nine percent of the calcium and phosphorus in the body is safeguarded in our bones. The utilization of a multi-nutrient daily supplement will give the prescribed day by day requirements of micronutrients. The main concern might be a slight rise in uric acid that can occur when fasting.

Noradrenaline

When we fast noradrenaline levels increase to give us the vitality to obtain more food sources (for our ancestors it would increase the ability to hunt and gather when they most needed nourishment). For example, 48 hours of fasting produces a 3.6% increase in the body metabolic rate, and not the dreaded metabolic 'shut-down' in response to a 4-day quick. In fasting regiments resting metabolism increase by up to 14%. It is fascinating that as opposed to easing back the metabolism, rather the body revs it up in response to fasting. Regimens involving calorie restriction, and/or avoidance of carbohydrates do not offer the advantages of fasting regimens that actually contribute to various hormonal adjustments that all have the earmarks of being profoundly valuable to our wellbeing on numerous levels. Fasting changes the body from consuming sugar to consuming fat. Resting metabolism isn't decreased, but rather improved.

Fat is our body's protected nourishment. Logically, it is clear that we are, consuming our body when we use our fat, and we are 'expanding' our fat when we store it. Studies show that the epinephrine (adrenalin) initiated fat consumption doesn't rely on reducing glucose. There are two ways to ingest energy, either sugar and fat. Sugar is glucose and chains of glucose (glycogen) are stored in the liver. Much like a refrigerator, where it is easy to put food in or take food out, there is only so much room for food in the space. Because it is easier to utilize, the body uses glucose first. Fat is nourishment that is protected for the longer periods of no intake, more like our freezer (rather than our refrigerator). It's harder to prepare food from the freezer and you have to have time to take it out and prepare it, yet the extra room and the time it can remain there are both very helpful for storing it. Our concern for weight reduction is how to get out the energy we've put in the body's equivalent to the freezer compartment. If our body is continuously acclimated to consuming sugar, it won't easily access fat for energy consumption. Even though there is more than enough 'food' safeguarded as fat in the 'freezer,' we feel hungry. One arrangement is to exhaust out the freezer by Fasting. This way permits us to effortlessly get into the nourishment in the freezer and consume fat. Fasting gives us a simple method to get at our fat stores.

Chapter 7. Different types of Intermittent Fasting

Part one

Intermittent Fasting has been very popular in the recent years. It's touted as a method of weight loss, improving metabolism, and possibly even extending our lifespan. Not unexpectedly, and due to its popularity, many different kinds of intermittent fasting processes have been developed.

There are six well-known methods of doing intermittent Fasting.

- The 16/8 intermittent fasting: Fasting for 16 hours every day
- The 5:2 Intermittent Fasting: Fasting for two days in a week
- Eat-Stop-Eat: fasting for 24-hour once or twice a week
- Alternate-day fasting: Fast after one day
- The Warrior Diet: Fasting in the day, eat more at night
- Spontaneous meal skipping: Skip meals when you can

The 16/8 intermittent fasting: Fasting for 16 hours Everyday

16:8 Fasting that people also call the 16:8 eating routine or 16:8 course of action, is a particular type of Fasting. People who follow this eating plan will do Fasting for 16 hours every day and consume the sum of their calories in the remaining 8 hours.

Advantages of the 16:8 arrangement incorporate weight reduction and fat reduction and the anticipation reduction of type 2 diabetes and other obesity-related conditions. A few people accept that this technique works by supporting the body's circadian rhythm, its internal clock. Many people who follow the 16:8 meal plan keep away from foods from evening time and for part of the morning all night. They will, in general, consume their daily calories during the middle of the day. There are no limitations on the sorts of food measures that an individual can eat during the 8-hour window. This adaptability makes the arrangement generally simple to follow.

The most effective way to do it:

The least demanding approach to follow the 16:8 eating routine is to pick a 16-hour fasting window that incorporates the time an individual spends resting. A few specialists suggest completing food utilization in the early night, as digestion eases back down after this time. A few people will most likely be unable to consume their evening dinner until 7 p.m. or, even, later. It is ideal to stay away from eating for 2–3 hours before bed. People may pick one of the suggested 8-hour eating windows: 9 a.m. to 5 p.m. 10 a.m. to 6 p.m. Noon to 8 p.m. Inside this period, individuals can eat their dinners and snacks on the right occasions that suit them. Eating routinely is essential to control glucose peaks and valleys and to control appetite. A few people may need to locate the best eating window and eating times for their way of life.

Recommendations for 16:8 Intermittent Fasting:

While the 16:8 irregular fasting plan doesn't indicate which things to eat and keep away from, it is great to concentrate on healthful eating and restrict or maintain avoid consuming junk food. The utilization of an excess of unhealthful eating may cause weight gain and increase your risk of illness. A well-balanced eating routine focuses on:

Fruits and vegetables, which can be fresh, frozen, or canned (in water)

Whole grains, including quinoa, darker rice, oats, and grains

Lean protein sources include poultry, fish, beans, lentils, tofu, nuts, seeds, low-fat curds, and eggs.

Healthful fats from fatty fish, olives, olive oil, coconuts, avocados, nuts, and seeds.

Natural products, vegetables, and whole grains are high in fiber to help keep an us feel full satisfied for longer periods of time. Fortifying fats and proteins can likewise add to satiety.

Drinking water routinely throughout for the day can help decrease calorie consumption since individuals frequently confuse thirst for hunger. The 16:8 eating routine arrangement allows non-calorie drinks, for example, water, unsweetened tea, and espresso — during the 16-hour fasting window. It is imperative to have liquids routinely to avoid dehydration.

Instructions:

Individuals may think that it's simpler to adhere to the 16:8 eating routine when they follow these guidelines: Drinking homegrown cinnamon tea during the fasting time frame, as it might mask their hunger, consuming water generally throughout the day, watching less TV (to lessen exposure to pictures of food, which may activate our hunger). It is also suggested that avoid exercise during before or during the eating window, as exercise can trigger hunger. Practicing careful eating while eating dinners and trying meditation during the fasting time frame to permit cravings for food to pass.

Medical Advantages:

Scientists have been studying intermittent Fasting for a considerable length of time. These studies on irregular Fasting, including 16:8 Fasting, demonstrates that it might give the following advantages:

Weight reduction and fat loss:

Eating during a set period can assist individuals with decreasing the number of calories that they eat. It might likewise help support digestion. A recent report suggests that intermittent Fasting prompts more substantial weight reduction and fat loss in men with stoutness than the customary calorie limitation does. Research from 2016 reports that men who followed a 16:8 methodology for about two months, compared with men who didn't, indicated a decrease in fat mass. These other participants didn't keep up their muscle mass.

Interestingly, a recent report discovered almost no distinction in weight reduction between participants who tried irregular Fasting, as alternating day fasting compared to 16:8 Fasting, and the individuals who decreased their general calorie admission. The dropout rate was additionally high among those in the irregular fasting group.

Other Disorders:

Supporters of intermittent Fasting propose that it prevents the development of health problems, including Type 2 diabetes, Heart Conditions, and some Neurodegenerative conditions.

A 2014 survey reports that irregular Fasting shows a guarantee for a decrease of type 2 diabetes and weight reduction in individuals who are obese or overweight, in contrast to customary calorie limitation. In any case, the analysts alert that more research is vital before they can arrive at concrete conclusions.

A recent report shows an 8-hour eating window may help decrease blood pressure in obese adults, notwithstanding the weight reduction. Different investigations report that intermittent Fasting diminishes fasting glucose by 3–6% in those with prediabetes, even though it has no impact on healthy individuals. Likewise, it might decrease fasting insulin by 11–57% following 3 to 24 weeks of irregular Fasting. Time-limited fasting, for example, the 16:8 technique, may also support learning and memory and hinder disorders that influence the cerebrum. A 2017 yearly audit noticed that animal studies have demonstrated that this type of Fasting diminishes the danger of nonalcoholic fatty liver and malignant growths.

Broadened life span:

These studies propose that intermittent Fasting may assist humans with living longer. For instance, one investigation found that intermittent Fasting expanded the life expectancy of female mice. The National Institute on Aging points out that, despite considerable research, scientists cannot clarify why Fasting may extend life span. Subsequently, they can't affirm the long term affects of such a regimen. Study with human subjects are restricted. The potential advantages of irregular Fasting for the human life span are not yet known.

Reactions and risks:

16:8 intermittent Fasting has some related risks and responses. Therefore, the regimen isn't recommended for everybody.

Potential symptoms and dangers include:

Hunger, low energy, and fatigue at the beginning of the plan; Overeating or unhealthful eating during the 8-hour eating window due to over increased cravings; Heartburn or gastric reflux because of overeating. Discontinuous Fasting might be less advantageous for women than men. Some studies on individuals recommends that intermittent Fasting could adversely influence female fertility.

People with a background marked by disorder eating may wish to avoid the use of Intermittent Fasting. The National Eating Disorders Association cautions that Fasting is a risk factor for dietary problems. The 16:8 regimen may likewise not be reasonable for those with a history of depression and anxiety. Some studies demonstrates that transient calorie limitation may calm moods, but that constant calorie limitations can have the opposite of worsening mood. More research is essential to comprehend the ramifications of these findings. 16:8 intermittent Fasting is not recommended for the individuals who are pregnant, breastfeeding, or attempting to get pregnant. The National Institute on Aging indicates that there is insufficient proof to suggest any fasting diet, particularly for more senior adults. Individuals who wish to try the 16:8 technique or different sorts of irregular Fasting should get advice from with primary care physician prior to initiating the regimen, particularly considering their use of medications and other health considerations: any individual who has any worries or encounters any negative impacts of an eating regimen should see a specialist. Conclusion: 16:8 intermittent Fasting is a mainstream type of Intermittent Fasting. Potential advantages incorporate weight reduction, fat loss, and a decrease in the danger of certain illnesses. This eating regimen plan may likewise be more straightforward to follow than other different types of Intermittent Fasting. Individuals doing 16:8 intermittent Fasting should concentrate on eating high fiber whole foods, and they should remain hydrated throughout. The 16/8 strategy includes day-by-day fasts of 16 hours for men and 14-15 hours for women. Every day, one limits intake to an 8-to 10-hour "eating window" where you can fit in 2, 3, or more meals.

The 5:2 Intermittent Fasting: Fasting for 2 Days in a week

The 5:2 eating routine consists of eating as usual five days of the week while limiting calories to 500-600 for two days out of the week. This eating regimen is likewise called The Fast Diet and was advanced by British writer Michael Mosley. On the fasting days, it is prescribes that woman eat 500 calories, and men eat 600 calories. For instance, you may eat regularly each day of the week except Mondays and Thursdays. You eat two little suppers (250 calories for every dinner for women instead of 300 calories for men). As critics accurately call attention to, no studies have tested the 5:2 eating routine itself. Yet, there are many studies on irregular fasting advantages.

BRIEF Description:

The 5:2 eating regimen, or the Fast eating routine, includes eating 500-600 calories for two days out of the week and eating the other five days as you usually would. Irregular Fasting is an eating design that provides for regular Fasting. The 5:2 eating regimen, otherwise called The Fast Diet, is the most well-known discontinuous fasting diet. British writer Michael Mosley advanced it. It's known as the 5:2 eating regimen for five days of the week are typical eating days, while the other two limit calories to 500–600 every day. Since there are no prerequisites about which particular foods to eat, but instead when you ought to eat them, this eating routine is, to a greater extent, a way of life.

The most effective method to do the 5:2 Diet:

For five days out of every week, you eat as you ordinarily would and don't need to consider limiting calories. On the other two days, you lessen your calorie intake to a fourth of your typical needs. This plan is around 500 calories consistently for women and 600 for men. You can pick whichever two days of the week you like, as long as there is, on any occasion, one non-fasting day between them. One primary method for arranging the week is to fast on Mondays and Thursdays, with a few little meals, and eat as you ordinarily would for the remainder of the week. Emphasize that eating "regularly" doesn't mean you can eat anything. Should you choose to gorge on low-quality nourishment; you most likely won't lose any weight, and you may even put on weight. You ought to eat a similar measure of nourishment as though you hadn't been fasting by any means.

The 5:2 eating regimen includes regularly eating for five days out of every week, at that point, confining your calorie admission to 500–600 calories on the other two days.

Medical Advantages of Intermittent Fasting:

There are not many examinations on the 5:2 eating routine specifically. Notwithstanding, many studies on intermittent Fasting have been done, which shows impressive medical advantages. One significant advantage is that intermittent Fasting is by all accounts simpler to follow than constant calorie limitation, for specific individuals. Additionally, numerous investigations have indicated that various sorts of irregular Fasting may essentially diminish insulin levels. One study demonstrated that the 5:2 eating regimen caused weight reduction much like ordinary calorie limitation. Also, the eating regimen was viable at decreasing insulin levels and improving insulin affectability. A few investigations have investigated the impacts of adjusted substitute day fasting, which is fundamentally the same as the 5:2 eating routine (essentially, it's a 4:3 eating regimen). The 4:3 eating routine may help lessen insulin resistance, asthma, occasional hypersensitivities, heart arrhythmias, menopausal hot flashes, and that's only the tip of the iceberg. One randomized controlled examination in both average weight and over-weight people indicated significant advantages in the group doing 4:3 Fasting, contrasted with the benchmark group that ate typically. Following 12 weeks, the fasting group had: reduced body weight by over 11 pounds (5 kg). Reduced fat mass by 7.7 pounds (3.5 kg), with no adjustment in bulk. Reduced blood levels of triglycerides by 20%. Increase LDL molecule size, which is a health benefit. Reduced levels of CRP, a significant marker of inflammation. Decreased levels of leptin by up to 40%. The 5:2 eating routine may have a few significant medical advantages, including weight reduction, diminished insulin resistance, and reduced inflammation. It might also improve blood lipids.

The 5:2 Diet for Weight Loss:

If you have to get thinner, the 5:2 eating regimen can be effective when done right. For the most part, this meal plan is because the 5:2 eating design encourages you to consume fewer calories. In this manner, it is significant not to make up for the fasting days by eating considerably more on the non-fasting days. Discontinuous fasting doesn't cause more weight reduction than customary calorie limitation if total calories coordinate. Fasting conventions like the 5:2 eating routine have demonstrated a great deal of success in weight reduction reviews: one review found that changed alternate day fasting prompted weight reduction of 3–8% through the span of 3–24 weeks. In a similar report, members lost 4–7% of their abdominal girth, implying that they lost a great deal of unhealthy stomach fat. Intermittent Fasting causes fewer decreases in bulk (or muscle mass) compared to weight reduction with customary calorie limitation.

Discontinuous fasting is even more effective when combined with fitness workouts. The 5:2 eating routine ought to be successful for weight reduction whenever it is done accurately. It might help lessen belly fat, just as helps to keep up muscle mass during weight loss.

Instructions for Eating on Fasting Days:

There is no standard for what or when to eat on fasting days. A few people find it works best by starting the day with a little breakfast, while others think that it's best to begin eating as late as could be allowed. By and large, there are two meal designs that individuals follow:

Three little meals: Usually breakfast, lunch, and supper

Two marginally larger meals: Only lunch and supper. Since calorie intake is constrained — 500 calories for women and 600 calories for men, it is advised to utilize your calories carefully. Attempt to concentrate on nutritious, high-fiber, high-protein nourishment that will cause you to feel full without absorbing a large number of calories. Soups are a great choice on fast days. Studies have demonstrated that they may cause you to feel full and satisfied with healthy nourishing, low calorie content. Here are a couple of instances of foods that might be appropriate for fast days: A liberal amount of vegetables, natural yogurt with berries, boiled or prepared eggs, grilled fish or lean meat, cauliflower rice, soups (for instance, miso, tomato, cauliflower, or vegetable), low-calorie cup soups, black espresso, tea, sparkling water.

Conclusion: There are numerous meal plans accessible on the web for 500–600 calorie fast days. Adhering to nutritious, high-fiber, and high-protein nourishments is a good choice.

Who Should Avoid the 5:2 Diet:

Though intermittent Fasting is ok for sound, all-around healthy individuals, it sometimes doesn't have a good effect on everybody. A few people ought to stay away from dietary limitations and fasting totally. These include individuals with a background marked by nutritional issues. Individuals who regularly experience drops in glucose levels, pregnant women, nursing moms, young people, children, and people with type 1 diabetes, as well as those who are malnourished, underweight, or have known nutritional insufficiencies. Any women are attempting to get pregnant or struggling with fertility issues.

Moreover, irregular Fasting may not be as useful for women as men. A few women have found that their menstrual period reduced or stopped while following this eating plan. Typically their cycles returned to normal when they came back to a usual eating routine. Due to these findings women should be cautious when beginning any type of intermittent Fasting and quit doing it quickly if any antagonistic effects occur.

Conclusion

The 5:2 eating routine is a simple, compelling approach to shed pounds and improve metabolic wellbeing. Numerous individuals think that it's a lot simpler to adhere to than an ordinary calorie-limited eating routine. In case you're hoping to get thinner or improve your wellbeing, the 5:2 eating routine is undoubtedly an exciting option.

Eat-Stop-Eat: Fasting for 24-hour
Once or twice a week

"Eat-Stop-Eat incorporates a 24-hour fasting, either more than once consistently." This strategy promoted by wellness master Brad Pilon and has been very mainstream for many years. It was created by Brad Pilon, writer of the mainstream and apropos titled book, "Eat Stop Eat." Pilon was motivated to compose this book after inquiring about the impacts of momentary Fasting on metabolic wellbeing at the University of Guelph in Ontario, Canada. Pilon explained the Eat-Stop-Eat technique isn't your average weight reduction diet. It's a method to re-examine what you have been recently educated about regarding supper timing and recurrence and how that connects with your health. By fasting from dinner one day to next one the following day, adds up to an entire 24-hour Fast. For instance, if you finish supper at 7 p.m. Monday and don't eat until supper at 7 p.m. the following day, you've accomplished an entire 24-hour fast. You can likewise fast from breakfast to breakfast or lunch to lunch. Each time it will be equivalent to 24 hours of fasting. Water, espresso, and other non-caloric drinks are permitted during Fasting, but no caloric foods are permitted. In case you're doing this to get thinner, it's significant that you eat regularly during the eating time frames. As in, eat a similar measure of nourishment as though you hadn't been fasting at all. The potential drawback of this strategy is that an entire 24-hour fast might be genuinely hard for some individuals. You don't have to jump in immediately, but rather beginning with 14-16 hours of fasting in a day and gradually increasing time from that point on is a reasonable way to adapt.

Conclusion

Eat-Stop-Eat is an irregular fasting program with a couple of 24-hour fasts every week. The idea of intermittent Fasting has taken the well-being and health world by storm. Early research proposes that taking part in occasional, transient fasting practices could be a critical and viable approach to shed unwanted weight and improve metabolic wellbeing. There are different approaches to executing an irregular fasting plan into your daily practice; however, the Eat Stop Eat strategy has become quite well known and effective.

Implementation of Eat stop eat Fasting:

Executing the Eat Stop Eat diet is quite clear. You pick a couple of non-back to back days out of every week during which you refrain from eating or fast for an entire 24-hour time frame. For the remaining 5–6 days of the week, you can eat as you like. However, it's prescribed that you settle on reasonable food decisions and abstain from consuming more than your body needs. Even though it doesn't intuitively appears to, you do actually eat something on each scheduled day of the week when utilizing the Eat Stop Eat technique. For example, in case you're fasting from 9 a.m. Tuesday until 9 a.m. Wednesday, you'll try to eat a dinner preceding 9 a.m. on Tuesday. Your next meal will happen after 9 a.m. on Wednesday. Along these guidelines, you guarantee you're fasting for an entire 24 hours; though, not longer.

Remember that even on long fasting stretches of Eat Stop Eat, legitimate hydration is a definite requirement. Drinking a lot of water is the best decision, but on the other hand, you're permitted different kinds of fluids without calories; for example, unsweetened or artificially sweetened coffee or tea. Eat Stop Eat is an irregular fasting diet that you fast for 24 hours a few times every week. Eat Stop Eat could prompt weight reduction due to specific metabolic movements when your body is in a fasting state. The body's favored fuel source is carbs. When you eat carbs, they're separated into a usable type of energy known as glucose. After about 12–36 hours of Fasting, the vast majority of people will consume the glucose they have stored in their bodies and change to utilizing fat as an energy source. This moment is a metabolic state known as ketosis. Early research proposes that due to this metabolic move, delayed Fasting may support fat use in a way that conventional eating of less junk food procedures cannot. Information on this potential advantage is restricted, and there is by all accounts huge fluctuations in how rapidly individuals change into a state of ketosis. Given this fact, it's improbable that everybody will arrive at ketosis inside the 24-hour fasting window utilized in the Eat Stop Eat diet. More research expects to see how metabolic changes on an Eat Stop Eat diet can impact fat loss and considerable weight reduction endeavors. Eat Stop Eat may bolster weight reduction through decreased calorie intake as well as metabolic changes. But results cannot be guaranteed to be the same for everybody. Eat Stop Eat Risks: Following are potentially harmful side aspects of the Eat Stop Eat diet.

Insufficient nutrient intake:

Specific individuals may struggle to meet the entirety of their nutritional needs on the Eat Stop Eat diet. With regards to slimming down, it's normal for individuals to consider nourishment as calories alone. But food is substantially more than calories. It's additionally a significant source of nutrients, minerals, and other helpful components that help your vital life sustaining function. Following Eat-Stop-Eat, individuals need to consider the nourishments they consume on their non-fasting days to guarantee sufficient protein, fiber, nutrient, and mineral intake all through their eating regimen. If you have exceptionally high dietary requirements for energy, you may struggle to consume enough to meet the body's needs. You may lose too much weight or you may have poor health due to a lack of other nutrients.

Low blood sugar:

A few people utilizing intermittent Fasting consume fewer calories like Eat- Stop-Eat to improve glucose control and insulin effectiveness. Most healthy individuals have no trouble keeping up glucose levels during the 24-hour fasting periods required on Eat-Stop-Eat, but that may not be the situation for everybody. For example, for those with diabetes, broadened periods without nourishment may add to risky glucose drops that could be hazardous for specific individuals. If you take medications to manage your glucose or have any ailments that cause low glucose, you must check with your medical practitioner before you start the Eat-Stop-Eat or any other eating regimen that incorporates Fasting.

Hormonal change

Fasting practiced on the Eat-Stop-Eat Diet may add to changes in metabolic and conceptive hormone creation. The particular health changes that arise because of such hormonal changes are hard to foresee because of an absence of human research. A few studies propose that specific hormonal changes may offer positive medical advantages, for example, improved fertility. In contrast, others demonstrate a potential risk for negative impacts like insufficient regenerative hormone creation and pregnancy inconveniences. As a result of the blended information and constrained complete proof, Eat-Stop-Eat isn't, for the most part, suggested for any individual who's pregnant, breastfeeding, or intending to become pregnant. Furthermore, if you have a background marked by hormonal irregularity, sporadic periods, or amenorrhea, consult your doctor before beginning an Eat-Stop-Eat diet.

The psychological impact of Restrictive Eating:

While many of us report feeling a lot of dietary freedom while utilizing fasting as a weight loss aid, such consumption patterns' restrictive nature may negatively impact some individuals. Some analysis indicates that short-term fasts might cause irritability, volatile moods, and reduced desire. That said, proponents of intermittent fasts usually say that mood problems resolve when you have become aware of your fasting routine — although these claims haven't been formally tested. Restrictive Diets might also contribute to existing disordered eating behaviors, like bingeing or obsessional thoughts concerning food and weight. Because of this, Eat-Stop-Eat isn't for people suffering from disordered eating or an inclination toward developing these behaviors.

Conclusion: Eat Stop Eat could be a typical kind of periodic abstinence during which you fast for twenty-four hours once or twice per week. Research on this specific ingestion pattern is limited; however, it does support weight loss by reducing calorie intake and changes in metabolic activities that favor fat loss. Nevertheless, no specific results may be guaranteed. Though abstinence is usually considered as safe, it might have adverse effects like inadequate nutrient intake and low glucose, therefore developing unhealthy digestion patterns. As always, consult your physician if you're unsure whether or not Eat-Stop-Eat is an appropriate weight loss strategy for you.

Chapter 8. Alternate-Day Fasting: Fast After One Day

Part two

Alternate-Day Fasting is another technique to incorporate intermittent fasting into your lifestyle. You fast each alternative day on this diet, but eat whatever you wish when it is allowed. The standard version of this Diet involves "modified" Fasting, where you'll be able to eat five hundred calories on fast days. Alternate-day fasting (ADF) can be a powerful weight-loss tool. It will lower your risk for cardiovascular disease and sort out polygenic disorder.

How to do alternate-day Fasting: Alternate-day Fasting (ADF) is an intermittent abstinence approach. The basic plan is that you only fast on some days, so eat what you wish on the other days. This way, you merely have to be restrictive of what you eat 1/2 the time. On fast days, you're allowed to drink as many calorie-free beverages as you wish. Examples include water unsweetened coffee and tea. Suppose you're following an adapted ADF approach. In that case, you're additionally entitled to eat an additional five hundred calories on fast days, or 20–25% of your daily energy needs.

The most well-liked version of this Diet is named "The each alternative Day Diet" by Dr. Krista Varady. She conjointly did most of the studies on ADF. The health and weight loss advantages appear to be constant despite whether or not the fasting-day calories are consumed at lunch or dinner or as tiny meals throughout the day. Studies show that several individuals noticed alternate-day fast was abundantly more straightforward to maintain rather than the old style, everyday calorie restriction. Most of the alternate-day studies quickly adopted the adapted version, with five hundred calories on fast days. This fact can be thought-about far more than doing full fasts on abstinence days; however, it's even as effective.

SUMMARY: Alternate-day abstinence cycles between abstinence and regular intake; the leading popular version permits five hundred calories on abstinence days.

Alternate-day Fasting and weight loss:

ADF is very efficient for weight reduction. Studies of adults who are obese have a noticeable fat weight reduction of 3-8% of body weight in 2–12 weeks. Remarkably, ADF appears to be specifically beneficial for weight reduction among middle-aged people. Studies have explained that ADF and everyday calorie limitation are evenly helpful at decreasing dangerous belly fat and girth markers in people with obesity. Additionally, a 2016 analytical report revealed that ADF might be better than daily calorie limitation diets. It's simpler to follow, creates better fat reduction, and maintains extra muscle mass. Moreover, joining ADF with endurance exercise may create twice as much weight loss than ADF alone and six times as much weight reduction as endurance exercise alone.

ADF appears to be evenly beneficial regarding meeting diet needs, whether used with a high-fat or low-fat diet. ADF is very helpful for weight reduction and simpler to do than purely caloric limitation.

Alternate-day fasting (ADF) and body constitution:

ADF is said to have distinctive influences on body composition, both while you're dieting and during your weight-maintenance period. Reports analyzing daily calorie-limited diets in comparison with ADF clarify that they're evenly as advantageous at reducing weight and fat mass. Moreover, ADF results are extra beneficial at conserving muscle mass. This fact is essential, as reducing muscle mass with fat reduces the number of calories your body routinely expends, even at rest. One randomized controlled study analyzed ADF to a traditional, calorie-limited diet with a 400-calorie deficit. After an 8-week period and 24 unverified weeks, no differences were observed in weight recovery among the groups. However, after the 24 unconfirmed weeks, the ADF group had maintained more bulk and less additional fat mass than the calorie-restricted group.

Health advantages of alternate-day Fasting:

ADF has many health benefits.

Type 2 diabetes: Type 2 diabetes is responsible for 90–95% of diabetes cases in the United States. More than a third of Americans have prediabetes, a problem in which blood sugar levels are irregular, but not sufficient to be termed diabetes. Reducing weight and limiting calories is usually beneficial to improve or even reverse many signs of type 2 diabetes. Much like continuous calorie limitation, ADF shows a some risks for individuals with type 2 diabetes, especially those who are obese or overweight. However, ADF results do show the most beneficial effect in decreasing insulin levels and decreasing insulin resistance while improving blood sugar management. Having high insulin levels (hyperinsulinemia) has been connected to obesity and chronic diseases, such as heart disease and cancer. Among people with prediabetes, 8–12 weeks of ADF have been shown to reduce fasting insulin by about 20–31%. A decrease in insulin levels and insulin resistance may result in a significantly decreased risk for developing type 2 diabetes, particularly when combined with weight reduction.

Heart health: Cardiovascular disorders are the main cause of death globally, accountable for about 1 in 4 deaths. Several reports have explained that ADF is a better choice for overweight people and those with obesity to reduce weight and decrease risks and symptoms of heart disease. A study over 8–12 weeks including those who were overweight and those identified with obesity. The more combined health improvements included decreased waist circumference (2–2.8 in or 5–7 cm); Reduced blood pressure; Decreased overall LDL cholesterol (20–25%), which included more of the larger LDL-particles and a decrease in the hazardous small, dense LDL elements; Reduced blood triglycerides (up to 30%).

Alternate-day Fasting and Autophagy: One of the more beneficial influences of fasting on the body is the activation of autophagy. "Autophagy is a method where antiquated pieces of cells are destroyed and reprocessed. It is beneficial in halting ailments like a malignant cell growth, neurodegeneration, and coronary illness, and diseases." Animal studies have repeatedly revealed that both long-term and short-term fasting enhance autophagy and are connected to postponement in signs of aging and decreased risk of developing tumors. Moreover, fasting has been found to encourage longer life spans in rodents, flies, yeasts, and worms. Furthermore, cell studies have explained that fasting activates autophagy, resulting in a healthy and expanding life span. This fact has been verified by a human observational study where ADF diets decreased oxidative cell destruction and developed alterations that may be connected to a longer life span.

What to eat and drink on Alternate day fasting: There are no strict rules on what you can consume or drink on fasting days, except that your total calorie consumption shouldn't be above

500 calories. It's excellent to consume low-calorie or calorie-free drinks on fasting days, such as:

Water, coffee and tea. Most individuals think is best to consume one "big" meal late in the day. In contrast, others favor consuming their calories early in the day, or instead divide the calories between 2–3 small meals. Since these low calorie days involve strictly restricting your calorie consumption, it's important to focus on high-protein options and as well as low calorie vegetables. These options will give you a feeling of fullness without much caloric intake. Soups may also be a great choice on fasting days, as they manage to make you feel fuller than if you consumed the ingredients on their own. Here are some patterns of meals that are appropriate for fasting days:

Eggs and vegetables

Yogurt with berries

Grilled fish or lean meat with raw vegetables

Soup and a piece of fruit

A generous salad with lean meat

Conclusion

Alternate-day Fasting is a very beneficial method to reduce weight. It has a few advantages over conventional calorie-confined eating regimens. It's additionally shown to contribute to significant enhancements in numerous markers of physical wellbeing. Probably the best its numerous advantages is that it's shockingly simple to adhere to ADF regimens, because you just need to "diet" every other day.

The Warrior Diet

The Warrior Diet is one of the most popular types of the intermittent fasting regimens. This type of plan consists of fasting during the day and eating more at night. It does include the consumption of a small portion of raw fruits and vegetables during the day and then consuming one large meal at night, in a 4-hour window of time. Similar to the paleo diet, the Warrior Diet also suggests consuming particular foods, such as whole or unprocessed foods. Fasting, the lessening of, or the moderation of eating food, is a tradition that has existed from ancient to present times, and includes religious as well as health ideas. The Warrior Diet is a method of consuming foods that expands the cycles of time that we consume small amounts of food, with a short overeating gap. It has been developed as a beneficial means to reduce weight, increase energy levels as well as improve mental health. Some health specialists claim that this fasting technique is risky and not necessary. The Warrior Diet has been founded on records of the earliest warriors' ingestion patterns, who used small snacks in the day and then ate more at night. According to its developer, Dr. Hofmekler, it's pattern "improves the way we consume, feel, perform and look" by emphasizing the body through decreased food consumption, and thus triggering "survival instincts." People following this Diet fast for 20 hours per day, then eat as much food as they wish at night. In the 20-hour fasting time, people are encouraged to eat small amounts of dairy products, hard-boiled eggs, raw fruits and vegetables, and many non-calorie liquids. Importantly, 20 hours later, people can binge on any foods they wish in a four- hour over-consuming gap. Moreover, unprocessed, healthy, and organic food options are encouraged. Followers of the Warrior Diet argue that this procedure burns fat, improves concentration, enhance energy levels, and activates cellular repairs.

Weight Loss: Several intermittent fasting procedures, involving 20-hour fasting cycles, have been connected to weight reduction. One study of the Warrior Diet (fasting for 20 hours) discovered that people who ate meals over four hours in the evening lost more weight than those who ate a similar quantity of calories in meals throughout the day. Moreover, those who consumed one meal per day had significantly decreased fat and maintained more muscle mass. A new review of six studies concluded that many intermittent fasting forms, ranging from 3 to 12 months, were more effective at advancing weight reduction than no dietary intervention. Furthermore, though reducing calorie consumption is the widespread consequence of the Warrior Diet, some people who follow this pattern could eat too many calories in the four-hour eating duration and may experience weight gain.

Brain Health: The Warrior Diet is also getting more popular because of improvements noted in brain health. The Warrior Diet has been found to assist in the regulation of inflammatory pathways that affect brain function. Animal studies have explained that fasting lowers inflammatory markers like interleukin 6 (IL-6) and tumor necrosis factor-alpha (TNF-α) whose presence may harmfully influence memory and learning. Other studies demonstrated that fasting has a preventative effect on Alzheimer's disease. However, research on this aspect remains on-going. More human studies are needed to make conclusion on the importance of intermittent fasting on brain health.

Decrease Inflammation

Inflammation produced by oxidative stress is considered to be a significant factor influencing the development of various disorders like heart disease, diabetes, and particular cancers. It has been demonstrated that intermittent fasting may be an acceptable means to decrease inflammation in the body. One study in 34 healthy men explained that the 16:8 intermittent Fasting reduced TNF-α and interleukin one beta (IL-1β), which promote inflammation. A study in 50 people explained that those fasting for the Muslim holiday of Ramadan had significantly fewer levels of the inflammatory markers IL-6, C-reactive protein (CRP), and homocysteine, in comparison with non-fasting individuals.

Improve Blood Sugar Control

Some reports show intermittent Fasting can improve blood sugar control in those with type 2 diabetes. The tests conducted on ten people with type 2 diabetes demonstrated that fasting for 18–20 hours a day significantly reduced body weight and significantly improved fasting and post-meal blood sugar levels. Although the decreasing of blood sugar levels in a safe way is critical, as hypoglycemia can be dangerous and cause serious complications. For this purpose, people with diabetes who are considering trying out intermittent Fasting should first discuss the plan with their doctor

.

Drawbacks of the Warrior Diet

The Warrior Diet's most understandable restrictions limit the time you may consume most of your calories to four hours a day. This plan can be tough for some to stick to, especially when taking part in regular social activities like going out to breakfast or lunch. While some people may think they feel best when eating minimal quantities of calories over 20 hours, others may find that this pattern of consumption is not right for their lifestyle. This type of intermittent fasting is unsuitable for various people, including: Children, women who are pregnant or nursing, people with type 1 diabetes, those with heart failure, or certain cancers high level athletes, people with dietary issues or a history of disordered eating and finally, those who are underweight. Furthermore, some research proposes that intermittent Fasting can affect women's hormones more than men's. Some may feel unpleasant side effects like insomnia, anxiety, missed periods, and reproductive health disturbances. It could cause disordered eating because it prescribes overeating, which could be problematic for numerous people. Though Ori Hofmekler says that one should stop eating "when you feel pleasantly satisfied," this may not translate into healthy consumption practices for everyone. The Warrior Diet could result in binging and purging behaviors, especially in subjects in the danger of developing disordered consumption. Binging on significant amounts of food may also lead to feelings of guilt and shame, which can negatively affect mental health and body image. Finally, the Warrior Diet may cause side effects, some of which could be extreme. Potential side effects involve fatigue, dizziness, low energy, light-headedness, anxiety, insomnia, extreme hunger, low blood sugar (hypoglycemia), constipation, fainting, irritability, hormonal imbalance, and weight gain. Moreover, various health professionals claim that dieters will not get sufficient nutrients when following an intermittent fasting plan like the Warrior Diet. Adding supplements, choosing foods are dense with nourishments and ensuring calorie needs are met; vitamin prerequisites must be ensured by reasonably planning your nutrient intake when following the Warrior Diet.

How to Follow the Warrior Diet

Hofmekler proposes that anybody beginning the Warrior Diet should follow an exceptional three-week, three-arranged plan to "improve the body's capacity for using fat for essentials."

Phase I (week one):

"Detox." For 20 hours in the day, incorporate vegetable juices, clear juices, dairy (yogurt, curds), eggs, unrefined foods, as well as organic raw fruits and vegetables. In the four-hour overeating period, consume a salad with oil and vinegar dressing, followed by one large or multiple small feasts of plant proteins(beans), wheat-free whole grains, small amounts of cheese, and cooked vegetables. Coffee, tea, water, and limited quantities of milk can be consumed for the day. Phase II (week two): "High Fat." Over 20 hours of the day consume vegetable juices, clear broth, dairy (yogurt, cottage cheese), hard-boiled eggs, and raw fruits and vegetables. In the evening, in the four-hour of the overeating period, eat a salad with oil and vinegar dressing, followed by lean animal protein, cooked vegetables, and at least one handful of nuts. No grains or starches are consumed during stage II.

Phase III (week three): "Concluding Fat Loss."

The cycles of this stage consist of periods of high carb and high protein consumption.

Alternating between 1–2 days more in carbs; 1–2 days more in protein and less in carbs; 1–2 days more in carbs; and 1–2 days more in protein and less in carbs.

On high-carb days:

Over 20 hours of the day consume vegetable juices, clear stock, dairy (yogurt, curds), hard- eggs, and raw organic foods. In the four-hour feasting period, consume a serving of mixed greens with oil and vinegar dressing, followed by cooked vegetables, modest quantities of animal protein, and one principle starch, such as corn, potatoes, and pasta, grain or oats.

On high-protein, low-carb days:

Over 20 hours of the day consume vegetable juices, clear broth/stock, dairy (yogurt, curds), hard-boiled eggs, and raw organic foods. In the four-hour eating period at night, eat a serving of mixed greens with oil and vinegar dressing, followed by 8–16 ounces (227–454 grams) of animal protein with a side of cooked, non-starchy vegetables. Though grains or starches are not eaten during the phase-III feasting period, a little fresh tropical fruit can be eaten for dessert. Hofmekler urges that once people have finished the three phases, they should begin again from the earliest stage. As opposed to reencountering the complete cycle, you may, in like manner, miss the necessary settings and keep the principles of eating for 20 hours on low-calorie sustenance, followed by using substantial, protein-rich meals to fulfill yourself in the feasting stage. Serving sizes on the Warrior Diet are unclear, and there is no set calorie limitation. Hofmekler proposes the addition of daily multivitamins with different supplements like probiotics and amino acids as components of this eating regimen. People are also encouraged to engage in exercise, particularly involving strength and speed training, into their daily routines to enhance fat loss and also to stay hydrated with lots of water throughout the day.

What to Eat and What to Avoid:

Although people are permitted to eat any food they like, whole, nutritious, organic foods are encouraged. In addition, processed foods, preservatives, added sugars, and artificial sweeteners should be avoided. Foods to eat in small amount in the under-eating stage of the regimen:

Fruits: Apples, bananas, kiwi, mango, peach, pineapple, and so on.

Vegetable juices: beet, carrot, celery, etc. Broth: such as chicken, and beef. Vegetables: such as greens, carrots, peppers, and mushrooms.

Raw vegetables: Greens, carrots, peppers, mushrooms, onions, etc.

Condiments: Small amounts of olive oil, apple cider vinegar, etc.

Dairy: Milk, yogurt, cottage cheese, etc.

Protein: Hard-boiled or poached eggs

Drink: Water, coffee, tea

What you can eat in the overeating stage:

Cooked vegetables: Cauliflower, Brussels sprouts, zucchini, greens, so on.

Proteins: Chicken, steak, fish, turkey, eggs, so on.

Starches: beans, potatoes, corn, sweet potatoes, so on.

Grains: Oats, quinoa, pasta, bread, barley, so on.

Dairy: Milk, cheese, yogurt, so on.

Fats: Nuts, olive oil, so on.

Foods to avoid:

Candy

Cookies and cakes

Chips

Fast food

Fried foods

Processed meats (lunch meats, bacon)

Refined carbohydrates

Artificial sweeteners

Sweetened drinks like fruit juice and soda

Conclusion:

The Warrior Diet cycles 20 hours of little food consumption with four hours of overeating. Although there is little research promoting this specific form of Fasting, intermittent Fasting, in general, has been connected with many health advantages, from weight reduction to developing brain health. While some individuals may thrive on the Warrior Diet, others may think its rules too problematic to follow. This regimen of consumption isn't suitable for various people, like pregnant women and children. Though the Warrior Diet may be beneficial for many people, the tried and true method of eating healthy, enhancing activity, and reducing overall calories is something everybody can follow.

Spontaneous Meal Skipping

You don't need to follow an organized intermittent fasting plan to earn some benefits. Another choice is to easily avoid meals from time to time, for instance at times you do not feel hungry or ready to cook and eat. It's an illusion that individuals ought to eat every few hours, or they'll hit "starvation mode" or lose muscle. The physical body is well equipped to handle long periods of famine, including missing one or two meals from time to time. So, if you're not hungry at some point, skip breakfast and just eat a healthy lunch and dinner.

On the other hand, if you're away home and can't find anything you would like to eat, do a brief fast. It is possible to skip one or two meals at times you feel inclined to do so, and essentially these occasions create a spontaneous intermittent fast. Just ensure you eat healthy foods when you do eat meals.

General Conclusion on Fasting

There are plenty of individuals getting great results with a number of these aforementioned methods of incorporating fasting into their lives. Intermittent fasting isn't for everybody, nor is it something that everyone must do. It's just another tool within the toolbox, which will be useful for some people. There are reports that show that it's not going to be as beneficial for women as it is for men. It's also not going to be a recommended choice for people that have or are susceptible to eating disorders. If you choose to undertake intermittent fasting, it's important that you also generally make healthy food choices. It's impossible to binge on junk foods during the eating periods and expect to reduce and improve health. Calories, despite everything, should be checked, and nourishment quality remains important in our food choices. You don't need to follow structured intermittent fasting to decide to experience the benefits. Another option is to skip meals from time to time, such as times you don't feel hungry or are too busy. It's a myth that individuals must eat every few hours, or they'll hit "starvation mode" or lose muscle. The physical body is well equipped to handle long periods of famine, including missing one or two meals from time to time. So, if you're not hungry at some point, skip breakfast and just eat a healthy lunch and dinner. A spontaneous intermittent fast is skipping one or two meals once you feel inclined. Just maintain consumption of healthy foods during the times you do consume meals. Another more "natural" means to do intermittent fasting is to easily skip one or two meals once you do not feel hungry or do not have time to eat. There are vast numbers of people getting extraordinary outcomes with some of these fasting strategies. If you decide to embrace irregular fasting, be mindful that you choose a workable fasting regimen for your life. It's impractical to gorge on lousy nourishments during the times that you are eating and expect to decrease weight and improve wellbeing.

Chapter 9. Scheme Of Daily Diet

Discontinuous fasting is a style of eating wherein you go without food for a specific measure of time every day. To assist you with exploring your day, here's a manual for how to plan your dinners while fasting. Although this eating plan is organized around when you eat, what you eat is also significant. During the time frames when you're eating, you'll need to concentrate on good fats, clean protein, and starches from whole food sources.

Schedule Meals in Intermittent Fasting

While the thought of a fast may be overwhelming, especially if you haven't done it before, the intermittent short fast will genuinely be a great deal easier than several alternative kinds of eating plans. Once you begin your brief fast journey, you may notice that you feel fuller longer and might find the meals you will eat straightforward. There are some alternative ways you'll fast, as explained below. The combination of nutrients can offer you the energy you desire to boost your short fast advantages. Check what you will require considering any food intolerances, and use it as a guide for your specific health situation, and modify as needed from there. Remember, intermittent fasting doesn't essentially mean calorie-controlled; therefore, take care to eat in line with your caloric desires.

The essential Intermittent Fasting Meal Plan for Beginners

If you are new to fasting, starting by just eating for the longer period, from 8 a.m. to 6 p.m., is an excellent method to dunk your toes into the fasting waters. This arrangement permits you to eat each meal in addition to specific snacks, and at the same time, get in 14 hours of fasting inside a 24-hour window.

Breakfast: at 8 a.m., drink a Green Smoothie.

After fasting, start drinking a smoothie since it is somewhat more straightforward for the gut to process. You'll need to go for a green smoothie rather than a high-sugar natural product smoothie to avoid beginning your day on an exciting glucose ride. Include heaps of good fats to support your energy needs up until lunch!

Lunch: at noont, eat Grass-Fed Burgers.

Grass-fed organic burgers are a preferred midday meal during the week, and they are straight- forward to prepare. The burgers can be served on a bed of dark leafy greens with a dressing for supper are filled with B nutrients for solid methylation and detox pathways.

Dinner: at 5:30 p.m., eat Salmon and Veggies.

Salmon is an excellent source of omega-3 fats. Green veggies like kale and broccoli have high anti-oxidative properties. Other alternatives, to salmon, can be any wild-caught fish based on your personal preference. Serve a portion of your preferred vegetables cooked in coconut oil, and you have a simple superfood.

Chapter 10. Intermittent Fasting Meal Plan

With this regimen, you will eat just between the long periods of noon until 6 p.m. which leaves an entire 18 hours of fasting within 24 hours. Take a couple of cups of herbal tea to begin the day. Even though you are skipping breakfast, it's still essential to remain hydrated. Make sure to drink enough water throughout the day. You can likewise have herbal tea, (Most specialists concur that coffee, espresso and tea don't break your fast.) The compounds in tea have been found to improve the advantages of fasting by assisting and facilitating a decline in the appetite hormone ghrelin, so you can push through until lunch and not feel denied. Since you've expanded your fasting period an additional four hours, you have to ensure your first meal (around early afternoon) has enough good fats. The burger in the 8-to-6-window plan will function admirably, and you can include more fats in your dressing or top it with avocado! Nuts and seeds make an incredible snack that is high-fat and can be eaten around 2:30 p.m. Consuming these can help kill naturally active catalysts like phytates that can add to stomach related issues. Have dinner around 5:30 p.m., and remain in the 8-to-6-window plan, supper with a wild-caught fish or another clean protein source with vegetables is an incredible alternative.

First meal, midnight: Grass-fed burger with cheddar cheese

Bite, 2:30 p.m.: Nuts and seeds

Second meal: 5:30 p.m. Salmon and veggies

The changed 2-day supper plan: For this arrangement, eat clean for five days of the week (you can pick whatever days you prefer). On the other two days, confine your calories to close to 700 every day. Calorie limitation opens a considerable similar advantages to fasting for a whole day. On your non-fasting days, you'll have to ensure you're getting in good fats, clean meats, vegetables, and natural, unprocessed products. You can structure your dinners anyway it best works for you. On restricting days, you can have smaller suppers or snacks for the day or you can have a moderate-size lunch and supper and fast toward the beginning of the day and after supper. Focus on good fats, clean meats, and produce.

The 5-2 supper plan: You'll eat clean five days of the week on this arrangement but won't eat anything for two non-consecutive days of the week. For instance, you can fast on Monday and Thursday, and eat clean dinners on different days.

Nourishment on these five days will look simply like the remainder of the fasting plans—good fats, clean meat sources, vegetables, and some natural products. Remember that this arrangement isn't for beginners. You should speak with your primary care physician before beginning any fasting routine, particularly if you are taking medications or have a health condition. It is suggested that espresso or coffee consumers keep up their morning espresso consumption and that everybody who does fast remains appropriately hydrated.

Monday: Fast.

Tuesday: Eat good fats, clean meat sources, vegetables, and some organic products.

Wednesday: Eat good fats, clean meat sources, vegetables, and some organic products.

Thursday: Fast.

Friday: Eat good fats, clean meat sources, vegetables, and some organic products.

Saturday: Eat good fats, clean meat sources, vegetables, and some organic products.

Alternate day fasting

Even though this regimen is advanced, it's key is to try not to eat anything every other day. On non-fasting days, choose to eat good fats, clean meat sources, vegetables, and some natural products. Afterward, you can consume water, herbal tea, and reasonable serving of dark coffee, espresso or tea on your fasting days.

Monday: Eat good fats, clean meat sources, vegetables, and some natural products.

Tuesday: Fast.

Wednesday: Eat good fats, clean meat sources, vegetables, and some natural products.

Thursday: Fast.

Friday: Eat good fats, clean meat sources, vegetables, and some natural products.

Saturday: Fast.

Sunday: Eat good fats, clean meat sources, vegetables, and some natural products. You should know precisely how to plan suppers when beginning an irregular fasting plan. And keeping in mind that it may be challenging in the beginning when you start fasting, eventually it will feel natural and fit pretty seamlessly into your routine. In any case, start gradually and slowly, bit by bit, work up to further developed plans. It's likewise essential to recall that you may have some "off" days when irregular fasting doesn't work for you. Tune in to your body. If you have to eat outside of your usual eating window, it's OK, you can restart your fasting routine when you're feeling better!.

Chapter 11. Recipes

1) Eggs and grilled chicken on toast

Ingredients:

- 60 g chicken slices
- Two medium eggs
- 100 g baby leaf spinach
- Two slice toast
- Sea salt
- Black pepper
- 1 tbsp olive oil

Recipe

Marinate the chicken slices with salt, pepper, and olive oil. Then grill the chicken on the bbg or in a hot pan.

Stir-fry the spinach with olive oil and season with salt and pepper.

Beat the eggs and then cook in a pan with oil for 2 to 3 mins.

Toast the slices of bread. Prepare then the plate with one piece of toasted bread, the chicken, the scrambled eggs, the spinach, and cover with the second slice of bread.

2) Fruits sandwich

Ingredients

- 2 slices brown bread
- 2 tbsp peanut butter
- One strawberry
- One banana
- 1 tsp cinnamon
- Lemon juice

Recipe

Cut all the fruits into small pieces, mix them in a bowl with cinnamon and lemon, and let the flavours mix well. Toast two slices of bread on a hot plate. Serve the toasted bread with peanut butter and cover it with the seasoned fruits.

3) Chicken Corn Soup

Ingredients

- 50 g chicken
- ½ cup of corn
- ½ onion
- ½ cup tomato
- 1 tsp salt
- 1 tsp black pepper
- ¼ tsp Coriander
- 2 tsp Olive oil

- 1 cup of Water

Recipe

Put the oil in the pan and lightly fry the onions with the chicken cut into small pieces. Then add the corn and season with salt and pepper. Add the tomato and water and cook for 20 minutes. Adjust the salt, pepper, and add coriander. Serve the soup in a cup.

4) Spicy Tomato Soup

Ingredients

- 1 cup tomato
- One garlic clove
- 1 tsp salt
- 1 tsp black pepper
- ½ cup onion
- Olive oil 1 tbsp

Recipes

Grind tomato and, in the meantime, heat the olive oil in a pan. Next, add garlic clove and onion. Cook for 1 min and then add the spices. Then insert the tomato and add some water and cook for 3 to 4 minutes.

5) Chicken Soup

Ingredients

- 4 oz skinless chicken breasts
- Two medium carrot
- 3 tbsp chicken broth
- 2 tbsp rice vinegar
- 1 tbsp soya sauce
- 2 to 3 tsp salt
- 1/4 tsp black pepper
- 1 cup of water
- 1 cup peas

Recipes

Combine liquids and bring to a boil, cut chicken into pieces, add to broth mix, cut all veggies add in with the chicken and cook. Then add all ingredients and boil. When cooked properly, serve in a bowl and enjoy.

6) Green soup

Ingredients

For the soup:

- 2 tbsp olive oil (30 ml)
- One yellow onion (150 g)
- Three cloves garlic, minced
- 150 g fresh baby spinach

- 250 g dark leaf kale
- 137 g chopped broccoli
- 107 g chopped cauliflower
- 1/4 tsp cinnamon
- 1.2 L chicken stock or vegetable stock
- 25 g almond milk
- 1 tbsp fresh lemon juice
- 30 ml heavy whipping cream
- salt
- black pepper

For the topping:

- 1 tbsp olive oil
- 160 g halloumi cheese, diced
- 60 ml heavy whipping cream
- 60 g pesto

Recipe

Heat the olive oil in a soup pot over medium heat and add the onion and garlic chopped. Cook for 5 minutes, or until it's soft. In the meantime, clean and cut the spinach and the kale. Add the chopped vegetables and stir fry them for 5-10 min. Then add the broth and salt and pepper. Let the mixture cook for 15-20 min. Finally, season the soup with lemon juice, cinnamon, the whipped cream, and almond milk. In a small bowl, mix one tbsp of olive oil, the grated halloumi cheese, the whipping cream, and the pesto. Transfer the green soup in small individual bowls and season on the top with the pesto topping.

7) Vegetable soup

Ingredients

- 2 tbsp extra virgin olive oil
- One large onion, diced
- Three cloves garlic, minced
- Three medium carrots, diced
- Three celery stacks
- Two potatoes
- 2 tsp aromatic Italian mix herbs
- 4 cups vegetable broth and 1 cup water
- 2–15 oz can diced tomatoes
- One can of corn
- One can make kidney beans
- One bay leaf
- ¼ cup parsley
- 1 tbsp lemon
- juice
- salt
- black pepper

Recipe

Heat oil in a large pan at medium-low heat. Then add onion, garlic, and a teaspoon salt and cook for about 8 minutes. Next, add carrots, celery, potatoes, chopped before, and cook for five more minutes, stirring. Add the aromatic mix and cook for one more minute. Put the broth, water, tomatoes, corn, beans, bay leaf, and season with pepper.

Let the soup boil and then reduce the heat and let it cook for 35 min covered. In the end, add in parsley and lemon juice and season with salt and pepper. Serve in a bowl with crostini.

8) Avocado and Corn salad

Ingredients

- 1 cup of corn
- Two avocados
- ½ cup onion
- 1/2 cup tomato
- Two lemons,
- 1 tsp olive oil
- Salt (as needed)
- 1 tsp black pepper

Recipe

Boil corn or you can grill it. Cut all vegetables. Mix all these ingredients in a bowl. Add spices and sprinkle lemon juice.

9) Scrambled eggs with spinach and salmon

Ingredients

- 100 g spinach
- Three eggs
- Three slices smoked salmon
- Salt and pepper
- 1 tsp chives
- 1 tbsp olive oil

Recipe

To prepare this meal, you can use freeze or fresh spinach. Put spinach in a pan with a tbsp of olive oil, season it with salt and pepper, and lightly stir fry. Then add to the spinach the eggs, remember to beat before adding, and cook it moving with a spoon.

Cook for 2-3 minutes and add salt and pepper if necessary, and season at the end with chives. Serve on a plate the scrambled eggs with spinach and add the slices of the smoked salmon.

10) Tuna Salad

Ingredients

- 120 g tuna
- 2 tbsp minced celery
- 1 tbsp julienne carrot
- Valerian salad

- 12 tsp onion
- 1 tsp parsley
- 1 tsp mustard
- 1 tsp black pepper
- 1 tbsp lemon juice

Recipe

Marinate tuna with the juice of lemon, olive oil for half an hour. Then cook tuna in a hot pan for 6 minutes for each part. Serve the tuna on a plate with a salad combined with slices of onion, celery, carrot, and the valerian and season with salts, pepper, and cover all with a sauce prepared with oil and mustard.

11) High protein and low-fat Mozzarella salad

Ingredients

- 100g high protein low-fat Mozzarella
- 1 Tomato
- Three leaves of Lettuce
- One cucumber
- 1tbsp salt
- One tbs olive oil

Recipe

Cut all the vegetables to prepare the salad and season with salt and olive oil. Serve in a bowl, mixing with Mozzarella cut into small pieces. Alternatively, you can serve the cut vegetables on a plate and season them with salt and olive oil, and then serve the mozzarella on the side.

12) Grilled Salmon with ginger

Ingredients

- 120 g salmon fillets
- 1 tsp dry garlic
- 1 tbsp lemon juice
- zest of one lemon
- 1 tsp ginger root
- 1 tbsp of soy sauce
- 1 tbsp olive oil

Recipe

Put the salmon in a bowl with olive oil, the soy sauce, juice, zest of lemon, ginger, and garlic, and leave it to marinate for half an hour. Then cook the salmon in a hot pan for 5 minutes for each part. Serve in a plate season with some oil and lemon and eat it with a fresh salad.

13) Grilled Zucchini

Ingredients

- 1 Zucchini
- 1 tbsp olive oil
- Salt

- Tsp Pepper
- Tsp mint

Recipe

Cut the zucchini lengthwise, into strips, dry the zucchini with a paper towel, and season it with salt. Heat a hot plate, and when hot, cook the zucchini for 3 min per side. Once plated, season the zucchini with olive oil, pepper, and the fresh mint leaves.

14) Salad with potato, mushroom, and lentil

Ingredients

For baked vegetables:

- 1–2 tbsp extra virgin olive oil
- Three medium potatoes
- 2 cups of mushrooms
- ½ cup of walnuts
- ¼ cup of Aromatic herbs, like rosemary, thyme, sage
- salt and pepper

For the salad:

- Two bunches kale chopped
- One can of cooked lentils

For the dressing:

- 2 tbsp olive oil

- ¼ cup of balsamic wine vinegar
- 2 tbsp water
- 1–2 tbsp Dijon mustard
- ½ cup chopped shallot
- ½ tsp salt
- ¼ pepper

Recipe

Cut the potatoes into a cube and season in a bowl with olive oil, rosemary, salt, and pepper. Preheat the oven to 400F. Put the potatoes in a baking tin in one layer. Then cook in the oven for 45 minutes (or until tender and brown).

Add sliced mushrooms and chopped walnuts and bake for another 10-15 minutes, or until everything is brown. Meanwhile, prepare the dressing. In a food processor, mix olive oil, the balsamic, water, the mustard, the shallot and salt, pepper, and blend all the ingredients well. Put the kale into a large bowl and season with the blended dressing. Let it sit for about a minute. Next, add lentils and the roasted potato mixture. Season with more salt and pepper if necessary.

15) Fruit shake of mixed Fruits

Ingredients

- One orange
- ¼ papaya

- ½ banana
- Three strawberries
- ice

Recipe

Squeeze the orange and cut the berries, papaya, and the banana into small piece. Use a mixer to prepare the shake, by adding the fruits, the orange juice, and ice inside, and blend until they become homogeneous. Serve the drink cold.

16) Detox Spinach Smoothie

Ingredients

One apple

One medium banana

1 cup spinach

lemon juice

1 tsp black pepper

Water

Recipe

Peel fruits and cut them all into small pieces. Then mix it in the blender with lemon juice and water.

Chapter 12. Exercise For Fun, Not As A Requirement

I've saved exercise for the latter half of the book because your diet is the number 1 thing you need to focus on to lose weight. It's where most of your effort should be directed. The reason for this is simply a matter of practicality. You could go for a 1-hour brisk walk or simply NOT EAT that 400-calorie bagel and cream cheese. Exercise is essential for our health and that goes without saying, but it's secondary to fat loss. But for me, I have found that walking helps me unwind, clear my head, and suppress my appetite. For that reason, I think walking is the best thing you can do to help with your weight loss efforts. I like to walk for 40-60 minutes around lunchtime while everyone is sitting on their ass eating. Another benefit is that if you walk while fasting, your body will be converting your stored body fat into the energy source for your walk. Goodbye, body fat! Remember, it isn't necessary for your fat loss efforts, so do it if you like to, or to give yourself some extra calories for some social plans you have that will involve eating later. Want to have that gin and tonic tonight but don't have the calories left for your deficit? Go for a 40-minute brisk walk!

Strength Training

This last point I won't go into too deeply, but it's essential. When you are on a fat loss diet, you will INEVITABLY lose muscle. Your body will be using a combination of fat and muscle protein for energy. You want to try to prevent your body from using too much muscle. You don't want to be a muscle-less skeleton. The best way to avoid this problem is to do some form of strength training. I'll let you decide what that could be, but for me, I like to keep it as simple as possible, and I think you should too. It means simple bodyweight calisthenics. No gym. Just push-ups, pull-ups, squats, dips, etc. Your body is all you need.

Should I exercise during the fast?

Exercising anytime and anywhere will not harm you, it will only help keep you trim and healthy. You could sit in the office and do your exercises, which could mean just flexing your arms around to keep the blood flowing. You could perform some squats on the train platform till the train arrives, or you could twist your waist slowly around when traveling in a bus or even turn your neck clockwise and anti-clockwise while standing at the bus stop.

These are just a few instances where you could loosen up a few muscles in your body, which are all exercises, indeed, which would help you in little ways to keep fit. So the question of whether exercising during intermittent fasting is good or bad does not arise in these situations. Still, you would need to think about it prudently before you would try a new exercise program. The first step would be to get yourself organized as far as your intermittent fasting schedule is concerned. You would need to plan out and do what is best for you with a program that works for you, especially if you are afflicted with any illnesses or joint diseases. Each of us has our peculiar traits, attributes, strengths, and weaknesses. Hence, before choosing to exercise, we need to look at these quirks and then conclude what is best for us as an individual. What you see on the television with all those gorgeous models exercising away promoting various equipment and muscle enhancing vitamins and boosters may not be for you. Trying them could have adverse effects if you are not geared for that sort of regime; hence it would be prudent to select what exercises are right for you and avoid what is not.

Therefore, getting your act together as far as your intermittent fasting is concerned would be your number one priority before you embark on an exercise regime. It would also be advisable to seek professional help starting a program, to ensure that you do not injure yourself in the process. Once you have decided on your intermittent fasting schedule and the related exercise program, it would be advisable to proceed step by step without rushing into anything. Once you are on the periodic fasting schedule, your body will undergo some adjusting during the first few days, and keeping an eye on how you manage that would be the priority. It will likely take a few days. With your body in a transition mode, it would be advisable to keep a close watch on yourself if you are on the intermittent fasting schedule for the first time.

First-timers to intermittent fasting may have to adjust to the new metabolic activities inside the body. Coping with it depends on each individual's personality and physical condition. A healthy individual should be able to ride the uncomfortable few days with ease. Still, the same cannot be said of another who has some health problems or other inherent issues. Everything depends on how the person adapts with the situation and how best they come out of it and ride the storm's first few days. The selection of the appropriate intermittent fasting schedule and practicing it will help you lose weight, which has been why this method has become very popular in such a short period. Maintaining all aspects of your fasting plan, continuing it with vigor, and especially selecting the right foods to be consumed while you are on the plan, will contribute to meeting the goals you have set for yourself on his health journey. If you set your sights on your objectives and have all of your metaphorical horses running in the same direction, then losing weight and achieving your plan are possible. The exercise regime you select should start with achievable activities, you should not attempt exercises that you are not comfortable with, though you may increase the difficulty as your comfort and abilities improve in time.

If you need to challenge anything, in particular, give it much thought and weigh the pros and the cons before trying your hand at it. Though exercise may be seen as the ultimate weapon we have to control our body weight or the dreaded obesity, we need to tread cautiously before we try anything because injury looms around the corner. If you do something that your body is not ready for yet, you could regret it later. There have been many such incidents. It is always better to know that prevention is better than cure. Once you injure yourself, even an awkward pull of a muscle, you could be out of action for a very long time. All exercises are not for everyone. Some options may be good for you; hence knowing what is right and wrong will be important for you to consider as you select what exercises you want to add to your lifestyle.

Exercises during intermittent fasting can keep the inside and the outside of your body, in perfect harmony. When that is achieved, you will have met your ultimate goal. Hence a planned intermittent fasting schedule coupled with an exercise regime to fit your abilities should help you join the thousands of others who have immensely benefitted from this lifestyle. Just losing weight isn't really enough, it is the healthy vitality that comes from being able to do all of the activities we enjoy doing with our body that really contributes to success. Figuring out the best exercises to do may add unnecessary stress to this process of change, ultimately be guided by your interests and enjoyment of activity. Intermittent fasting and an exercise regime should fit well together. To reap the optimum benefits, be prudent and responsible in your choices.

What can happen during the fast?

Intermittent fasting is beneficial to our bodies because in anything we do, even in battle, it is advantageous to change strategy if we imagine this change as beating an enemy. Surprise, change, deviation from accepted norms these tactics change situations on a battlefield. The same goes for our bodies. Suddenly and intermittently changing our standard food intake system requires the body to react to the new and unexpected situation, not only in metabolic activity, but in all of the related functions involving all our vital organs. Our bodies may not be our enemy, but we can implement specific strategies that would equate it to a certain extent of being similar to an "adversary in a battle to live." We need to implement innovative strategies because the body doesn't always do what we want it to.

We may like to eat plenty of sweets. Still, the body says otherwise and strikes us down with diabetes. We may also love to eat hamburgers, pizzas, doughnuts, and other junk foods, but our body says, No! To tackle our insubordinate and obstinate bodies, we may need to implement new and innovative strategies to ensure we remain the boss, or our bodies' owners, and not become at the mercy of the chronic conditions that develop when we are not in tune with our bodies. Our bodies tend to be obstinate, they get stuck in patterns that can become devastating. Despite the good food we eat, when our body is stuck it feels like it has turned against us, and we certainly don't feel balanced or in harmony. Hence, to get back to health we may need to stop pampering it. Our body may benefit from being denied the comfort of having three full meals a day, and all the other yummy foods we consume. Our bodies are not responding with gratitude for the easy, predictable intake we provide, but rather for some of us, in time the body inflicts us with limiting disease or illness. Hence, the time has now come for us to implement new strategies to ensure that we don't provide our body with unlimited access to food.

By practicing intermittent fasting, we deviate from accepted norms and strategically change our body's metabolic activity. This lets the body know that we are indeed in charge. We will control the food intake as and when we want. When we do this, the body is sure to hit back. We will immediately experience its wrath and whiplashes by way of dizziness, light-headedness, nausea, headaches, stomach cramps, mood changes, and many other varying problems: with the sudden loss of food into the system the body initially refuses to submit. This battle may persist for a few days, but if you go through the uncomfortable process it is what we need to endeavor to win the war with our adversary, in this case, our body, and ensure we take back control of ourselves. Once we have won the first foray into battle, we should enjoy the newfound freedom to eat when and what we want, but that does not mean that we should revert to food that would be detrimental to our health. Intermittent fasting accompanied by its advantages, goodness, and wellness supersedes any uncomfortable feelings you may experience in those first few days. There is strong scientific evidence to drive home the point that it has a use for our bodies.

Intermittent fasting could be seen as a strategy to ensure that we deviate from the perennial habit of consuming food in the same ways we have practiced, from birth, or even as a hereditary habit followed by our parents and their parents before that. When we stop habitually consuming food and skip a meal, the body will react and ensure that our blood sugar levels are maintained; if not, either a low or higher could send us into an irrecoverable "diabetic coma." What the body will do is it secretes more insulin to ensure that the blood sugar levels are maintained at the appropriate and optimum levels. The issue with fatty acids collected in our bodies in the most unlikely places increases our body weight considerably. When we practice intermittent fasting, "leucine," the enzyme that helps in breaking down or synthesizing protein that we take from our food when it is prevalent in our bodies, is ordered by the body to go and take all that fat that has collected in the body, synthesize it and use it to provide the energy the body needs to sustain itself.

These two processes are among many other significant changes that occur when we deny the regular food flow into our systems. It is a proven factor that these changes helps to rejuvenate most of our vital organs. Il is important to be mindful of some aspects and thus if you are not physically healthy it would be advisable to obtain medical advice before starting an intermittent fasting schedule. It would also be prudent not to fast too often, as that can become a new habit that the body adapts to, or become obstinate about. The brain is the most crucial organ in our body, the control center of the whole show. It is the brain that we need to keep guessing as to what we should be doing next as far as the food intake is concerned. If we keep the brain guessing, that is good for the body as it adapts to make the required adjustments in the system to ensure that the body carries on with the essential work. There should not be any fear that just because your body did not get food to lunch today, it will shut itself off and drop dead.

Chapter 13. Benefits of Intermittent Fasting For Over 50

What makes it harder to get in shape after age 50? As we age we encountered digestion problems, weak joints, and insomnia; and the risk for developing numerous illnesses increases. Simultaneously, losing fat, hazardous abdominal fat, can significantly lessen your risk for such medical problems as diabetes, coronary failures, and malignant growths. The discontinuous fasting diet for women over 50 could fill in as a virtual wellspring of youth regarding weight reduction and limiting the opportunity to develop common age-related diseases. The life duration enhances steadily as calorie consumption is reduced (until starvation) and the diet period. Curiously, intermittent fasting can also improve the duration of life, even when there is only a small or no general calorie consumption reduction. In particular, intermittent fasting is a meal plan with a decrease in meal frequency, such as every-other-day fasting. Similar to calorie reducing diets, intermittent fasting (IF) can prevent risk factors for diabetes and cardiovascular disease in rodents. Disorders accountable for mortality in rodents like cancers, diabetes, and kidney disorders are also delayed or eliminated by calorie reduction and intermittent fasting. A rising amount of physiological influence of CL (Caloric Limitation Diet) and IF that can influence the body's capabilities to enhance the duration of health as discovered in rodents, monkeys, and humans. Noticeable factors between these are the following:

- Enhanced insulin tolerance that ended in decreased plasma glucose and better glucose acceptance
- Decreased amount of oxidative damage as designated by reduced oxidative damage to proteins, lipids, and DNA
- Enhanced adaptation to many types of stress involving heat, oxidative and metabolic stresses
- Enhancement of immune functions.

The two principal theories for the aging influence of dietary limitation are the oxidative stress assumption and the stress resistance assumption. Because CL and some IF schedules include a decrease in energy consumption, rarer free radicals are created in the cells' mitochondria and, therefore, fewer oxidative damage to the cells. When maintained on a CL or an IF diet, individuals extending from yeast and worms to rats and mice display enhanced resistance to various altered forms of stressors. This influence with tension is related to the cells' improved strength in numerous reconstructed tissues and resistance to injury brought about by oxidative, genotoxic, and metabolic offenses. The maintenance of stress resistance applies to CL and IF around a variety of species and science delivers robust verification that this dietary limitation delays aging and contributes to extending life span.

Effect on Cardiovascular System

According to the World Health Organization, 17.9 million people die every year because of cardiovascular disorders, about one-third of all deaths. Those most affected are individuals over 45 years of age. The death rate varies in both genders in any predictions of life span. Between the ages of 45–59, men dominate, the statistics of death from heart disease, while after the age of 60, the rates for women increase. These dissimilarities are associated with the cardio defensive influence of estrogens in premenopausal women. External (or variable) internal (or invariable) risk factors contribute in complex and inter-related ways to the development of cardiovascular disorders. Clear our age, sex, and hereditary factors are out of our capacity to control, they are "invariable". While smoking addiction, being overweight, being sedentary, illnesses of lipid digestion, hypertension, diabetes, and unhealthy diets are more modifiable factors. The presence of at least two dangerous risk factors contributes to the probability of the disease occurring. Therapy for those who have suffered a heart attack or been diagnosed with cardiovascular diseases involves the modification of lifestyle habits, medication and at times out of necessity invasive treatment (such as surgery). If we reduce our bad habits these actions will contribute to a decrease in death and pathogenicity, specifically in individuals with undetected cardiovascular disease. With a healthy lifestyle, a balance exists, i.e., smoking cessation, enhancing physical activity, or assuring appropriate body weight, all of these actions contribute to decreases in the risk of cardiovascular disease. With increasing numbers of people affected by obesity in the world, diet modification is a significant changeable factor to improve health. Meals can be changed and aligned with a healthy Mediterranean diet. For instance, a good meal plan consists of a high presence of vegetables, fruit, fish, and only whole-grain bread. On the other hand proponents of this diet suggest we avoid eating animal protein, excessively salty foods (recommended daily salt intake less than 5 g), and drinking sweetened beverages. Also, the Mediterranean diet avoids the consumption of large amounts of alcohol. The consumption of spirits is a maximum of 10 g/day in women and 20 g/day in men. For various people, intermittent fasting is low restrictive compared with the conventional caloric limitation diet. It includes taking a typical, daily caloric consumption with the use of short, stringent calorie limitation. It is possible to consume meals within this diet only in a determined range of time, day, or week. There are two ways to follow the IF diet that is time-limited feeding and alternate-day fasting. The famous three types of IF are

- 16/8 method
- Eat-Stop-Eat
- The 5:2 diet

The first one, also called the Leangains protocol, consider skipping breakfast and eat only in eight hours of the day. Then this method includes 16 hours of fast and 8 hours when it is possible to eat. In a more severe methodology, the nutritional gap reduces to 4 hours. The 16:8 method is more popular and relatively easy to follow. The second one comprises 24 hours of fasting duration. Then one time, or two, a week, the meals are skipped for an entire day. The 5:2 method consists of consuming fewer calories, 500-600 calories, for two non-consecutive days but regularly eating for the other five days. Various studies of Intermittent fasting in both animals and humans verify the benefits in health and weight control. Moreover, IF decrease body weight and enhance cardio defense.

The cardio defense enhancement found in following the alternate-day fasting diet is possibly linked to a limitation of fat tissue (in particular fatty tissue around the organs), increased adiponectin levels, and decreased concentration of leptin low-density lipoprotein (LDL). Time-restricted feeding consists of consumption within a specific period of time. The protocol may alter according to individual choices and lifestyles and include the restriction of fasting for several hours (6-12 hours). This protocol may aid athletes to gain body mass for a specific sports performance. Moro et al. submitted a trial on 34 resistance-trained males to a time-restricted meal regimen compared to a control group. After eight weeks of this treatment, the IF testing group encountered a significant decrease in fat mass. The non-fat mass remained constant in both groups (control and tested group).

The researchers observed a reduction in the arm and thigh muscle cross-sectional. Leg press maximal strength increased significantly. Also, the values of blood glucose and insulin decreased significantly only in the IF group. Time-restricted feeding is usually done daily and does not require suggested restrictions. The fasting gap may be at nighttime. In that way, it can assist some people in preventing night eating and follow a natural rhythm.

Calorie restriction improves flow-mediated vasodilatation in obese human subjects, which is linked with a visible enhancement in insulin sensitivity, proposing a function for improved glucose metabolism in the beneficial influence of caloric limitation on the endothelial level. Mutually, the accessible data suggest that calorie limitation and Intermittent Fasting diets raise synaptic plasticity, improves the persistence of neurons, and enhances the number of neurons generated from stem cells. So we conclude that the dietary restraint contributes to reducing cardiovascular and cerebrovascular risk factors.

Caloric restriction and intermittent fasting have a positive effect on preventing various prevalent risk factors for cardiovascular disease and stroke. Individuals with insulin resistance (diminished glucose control) are generally linked with elevated levels of plasma glucose and insulin, and at increased of cardiovascular disorders and stroke. Testing CL or IF on Rodents and monkeys show increased insulin sensitivity, which would be predictable to reduce their hazard of diabetes and cardiovascular disease. Cardiovascular disease and stroke depend on high levels of low-density lipoprotein (LDL) and low levels of high-density lipoprotein (HDL). Reports on rodents, monkeys, and humans propose that CL can reduce LDL while increases HDL cholesterol levels. CL also reduces the levels of oxidative damage in the cardiovascular system, as described by diminished oxidative modifications of proteins and DNA as well as lower lipid peroxidation levels in the heart.

Moreover, the limitation of calories decreases inflammatory processes that probably causes atherosclerosis, as explained by lower levels of leukocytes and circulating tumor necrosis component levels. CL can reduce, by repressing atherosclerosis, the risk of cardiovascular illness and stroke. IF also restores cardiovascular adaptation to stress. For instance, when rats exposed to immobilization were on an IF diet, the amounts of stress produced showed increases in blood pressure (BP) and heart rate (HR). However, when the IF rats were compared to those in the control group (who we provided food whenever they wanted it) the IF rats blood pressure and heart rates were lower. In the IF rats BP and HR each returned to baseline levels more quickly following the conclusion of the stress inducing immobilization than that of the control rats. Rats on the IF diet revealed initiation of the stress-receptive neuroendocrine system with the accumulation of stress. However, rats on the IF diet adjusted faster to replicated stress testing, as explained by decreased corticosterone results analyzed and compared with those on the control diet. As described, the heart rate adaptation is enhanced in rats supported on IF and CL diets, which is evidence of another physiological alteration that we can expect to decrease the overall risk of cardiovascular mortality.

Data from the National Institute on Aging report proposes that CL lowers the occurrence of many disorders and lowers mortality. Concerning the cardiovascular system, studies with monkeys show lower body weights and reduced body fat. Similar alterations have been detected in human analysis. In a report of obese women, it is found that after eight weeks of CL, they found considerable drops in both systolic and diastolic BP, LDL cholesterol, and triglycerides levels. These changes are predictable in reducing the danger of cardiovascular disorder and stroke. Intermittent fasting also protects neurons and cardiac muscle cells resistance to ischemic damage. In an array of scientific findings, we have shown that intermittent fasting causes reduced stress on brain cells. The brain cells react to this low stress by increasing their capacity to respond more rigorously to stress. For example, studies on neurons in the brains of rats or mice on an IF routine found that they become extra resilient to being damaged by oxidative, metabolic, and excitotoxic damage (neurons damaged by high levels of neurotransmitters).

The dispensation of 2-deoxy-d-glucose (2DG; a non-metabolizable glucose analog) to rats, which mimics some CR (Calorie Restricted Diet) traits, also raises stress-resistant proteins in brain cells. The research proposed the probability that IF would enhance neurons' resistance to a stroke because other data have displayed that protective proteins can lower ischemic brain damage. Two groups of rats were subjected to a transitory middle cerebral artery obstruction (as a model of ischemic stroke). One group was on an IF regimen, the other were in the control group for diet (food available as desired). In the rats on the IF diet, they meaningfully reduced the quantity of ischemia related damage to brain cells in contrast with those on the control diet. This diet also reduced the number of brain cells destroyed by the stroke. IF results that contribute to definitive conclusions that the IF diet made for better quality health in rats.

Similar to IF's influences, when rats were retained for three weeks on a daily physical exercise routine and then faced with cerebral ischemia, the brain's level of damage was significantly reduced. The operational conclusion was advanced when compared with non-exercise control rats. Moreover, rats retained on a CL diet or subjected to physical exercise for ten weeks displayed decreased mortality and improved results following isoproterenol-produced myocardial infarction (heart attack).

Good Health Enhancement

All over the past, various societies had discovered the advantageous effects on health and general welfare of reducing food consumption for definite periods, either for religious motives or when food was rare. The first extensive systematic study, published by Mc Cay et al. in 1935, highlighted the restricted eating diets and their capability to expand lifespan. Mc

Cay explained that feeding rats with a diet comprising of edible cellulose dramatically expanded both the mean and maximum life-span in these animals. Many studies have verified this conclusion and extended it to mice and other species like fruit flies, nematodes, water fleas, spiders, and fish. So dietary changes affect lifespan and improve overall health at any time of our lives. We can achieve a predisposition to prevent illness or pathology. Modification of primary dietary routine, now known as a caloric limitation, is the most effective way of expanding the life-span of mammals without genetically changing them. In particular, intermittent fasting has also been explained to extend lifespan and have beneficial health effects.

Rodents upheld on calorie-limited diets are usually smaller and leaner. They have less body fat and smaller major organs than animals who eat "on demand". The smaller, learner rats are probably more active, which may be brought about by the need to search for food. The typical reduction in physical activity as animals age is not as notable in the calorie-limited animals. However, these animals are more susceptible to cold temperatures that affect death in small mammals.

Crucially, both caloric limitation and intermittent fasting can reduce the severity of critical factors for diseases such as diabetes and cardiovascular disease in rodents. In many studies, the occasional fasting routine ends in an approximately 20-30% reduction in caloric consumption over time. Rats maintained on this alternate day CL feeding routine for 2-4 months enhanced hippocampal neurons' resistance to chemically produced degeneration. This progressive impairment of hippocampal neurons is also related to striking learning and memory preservation in a water maze spatial learning task. Thus, these dietary routines could have an essential benefit for incapacitating and prevalent neurodegenerative disorders such as Alzheimer's, Huntington's, and Parkinson's diseases.

Intermittent Fasting Effect on Lipid Metabolism

Survival and maintenance of species amongst others depend on their accessibility to food. That is why living organisms have progressed with many adaptive procedures that permit them to live periods of starvation. Some microorganisms or animals in the periods where they do not have access to food are dormant; for example, yeasts stay in a stationary phase, while mammals use the liver and adipose tissue for sustenance. These set up an energy storeroom for them that permit them to live in periods of deprivation. Fats production is an essential mechanism of the human body. The fats' amount varied due to the body's conditions, and their role satisfied the organism's request. One of the essential functions is that of the stoppage and energy function.

The adipocytes (or fat cells) preserve energy. Under specific circumstances, the energy is discharged from them under the effect of the enzyme lipase. After the consumption of a meal, the amount of glucose in the body increases. Then within a few hours, it reverts to the same condition it was in before dinner. The amount of ketones is reduced because the glycogen stored in the liver is not reduced. Throughout the intermittent fasting diet, which consists of planned fasting periods, there are noticeable metabolic variations in the body. During the day, all food that is eaten in 6-8 hours period increases the glucose levels in about 6 hours after a meal but it remains low for the remaining 16 hours and thus until the next day. During the 6-8 hours in an eighteen hour fasting gap, ketones increased. The human body adjusts to such periods of fasting. In the feelings of hunger, adaptation processes start to increase energy. When glucose is consumed in a fasting period, the body begins to use ketones that are elevated due to fatty acid changes. Fatty acids and ketones develop the necessary resources of energy for your cells. This changeover is called intermittent metabolic switching (IMS) or glucose-ketone (G-to-K) switchover. While the body is not being fed, and your refraining from consuming food, the amount of glucose, your body's primary energy source, is reduced. Then your body consumes the glycogen stored in the liver, stimulating the reaction called gluconeogenesis.

Moreover, insulin and IGF-1 (insulin-like growth factor-1) levels decrease in the blood, and glucagon levels elevate. The lipolysis of the fatty acids produces triacylglycerol and diacylglycerol. These move to the liver cells, where they are changed into β-hydroxybutyrate (BHB) and acetoacetate (AcAc) in the β-oxidation reaction and are further freed into the blood and consumed as a source of energy for your body's cell, especially those cells in the brain. Such biochemical changes in the cellular and molecular adaptations of neuronal nets in the brain. As a result they develop functions that contribute to resistance to stress, injuries, and diseases. These biochemical alterations of lipids following intermittent fasting result in weight reduction and improved lipid parameters. According to studies by Surabhi Bhutani et al., during the episodes of alternate-day fasting for 2–3 weeks presented a decrease in body weight of 3%. Prolonged use of alternate-day fasting produces a reduction of 8% body weight and decreased fat mass in the abdominal cavity (around the organs). In addition, the levels of total cholesterol triglycerides and low-density cholesterol (LDL) molecular sizes decrease and all of these alterations reduce the risk of coronary heart disease.

The Influence of Intermittent Fasting on Inflammatory Biomarkers

Atherosclerosis is a significant risk of disease and death in both developed and developing countries.

This pathology's clinical symptoms are ischemic heart disease, peripheral artery disease, and ischemic stroke. It is accountable for severe myocardial infarction and cerebrovascular events. It is also responsible for most deaths resulting from cardiovascular causes in the world. Atherosclerosis is a chronic inflammatory disease in which atherosclerotic plaque forms in arterial vessels, which causes sclerosis (or hardening) of the walls and tightening of the arteries. One of the principal risk factors is related to the presence of high levels of low-density lipoproteins LDL. These levels stimulate an inflammatory response and adhesion to the endothelium of blood leukocytes, primarily the monocytes. These migrate to the inner membrane of the vessels and are changed into macrophages; stimulating cells to release factors that add to the smooth muscle cell migration from the medial to the inner walls. Vascular smooth muscle cells reproduce and release extracellular matrix proteins.

There is a further gathering of lipids both within cells as well as extracellularly. The majority of critical factors for cardiovascular diseases and aspects of atherosclerosis may be reduced, by intermittent fasting. Inflammation is an essential element of disease development. Inflammatory factors, such as homocysteine, and interleukin 6 (IL6), take part in atherosclerotic plaque development. The research conducted by Aksungar et al. verified the influence of fasting on decreasing the amount of these proinflammatory factors. Forty healthy volunteers with an average body mass index (BMI) joined their study. They fasted in Ramadan, and were compared with 28 participants with a similar BMI index, that did not fast. Venous blood was tested to analyze the concentration of the above-described proinflammatory factors and was obtained one week prior to the start of Ramadan, in the last week of fasting, and three weeks following the fast.

Adiponectin is a collagen-like plasma protein whose concentration reduces in the course of atherosclerosis, insulin resistance, diabetes, and coronary disease. The usage of the IF diet enhances the emission of adiponectin from adipocytes. There is an opposite association between plasma adiponectin levels and body weight. The Cambuli research involving 104 children with obesity. They compared adiponectin's initial concentration with the concentration examined after one year of the diet combined with enhanced physical activity. This concentration was improved by 245%. The increase in adiponectin concentration was comparative to the decrease in body weight. Adiponectin achieves its job by proceeding on adiponectin receptors realized in two isoforms, AdipoR1 AdipoR.

It displays anti-atherosclerotic and anti-inflammatory influences by inhibiting the adhesion of monocytes to endothelial cells. It also inhibits the emission of the vascular cell adhesion molecule 1 (VCAM-1), endothelial-leukocyte adhesion molecule 1 (ELAM-1), and intracellular adhesive molecule 1 (ICAM-1) on vascular endothelial cells. The study was proven by Ouchi et al. with in-vitro reports on individuals aortic endothelial cells incubated for 18 h in the presence of adiponectin. An adhesion assay assessed adhesion, produced by tumor necrosis element alpha (TNF-alpha), of THP-1 line monocytes to individuals' aortic endothelial cells. The appearance of the molecules was assessed by ELISA (enzyme-linked immunosorbent assay). The anti-atherosclerotic performance of adiponectin has been proven in several animal models and studies involving cell cultures. For example, reports organized by Okamoto et al., confirmed transcriptase-polymerase chain reaction (real-time) and ELISA testing, explained that adiponectin has an anti-inflammatory action in macrophages by inhibiting the creation of CXC 3 receptor chemokine ligands. In in-vivo reports on mice lacking in apolipoprotein E/adiponectin, there was an enhancement in IP-10in plasma, and enhanced deposition of T lymphocytes in blood vessels and atherosclerosis was analyzed to a single apoE deficiency. Matsuda et al. explained in adiponectin-lacking mice that a shortage of this protein enhances smooth muscle cells' propagation and relocation by increasing HB-EGF manifestation (heparin-binding epidermal growth element).

The IF diet has been linked with improved adiponectin levels and was proven in reports organized by Wan et al. These reports were carried out on rats allocated to groups with an ad-lib diet and IF for three months. Animals with an IF diet were denied food for 24h, every other day. The rats' left coronary artery was ligated to produce myocardial infarction. Animals with an IF diet had a tremendous amount of adiponectin, and the area of ischemia was smaller than those of the control group. Essentially lower inflammatory indexes were examined, while leukocytes and IL6 were analyzed in rats with an unrestricted diet. An essential hormone discharged by adipocytes is leptin. It has a pro-atherogenic influence. Levels were elevated in obese people and is correlated with body mass index (BMI), total cholesterol, triglycerides, blood pressure, and inflammation markers. These relationships were confirmed in reports by Sattar et al., in which leptin levels were built up in 550 men with lethal coronary illness (deadly CHD) or nonfatal myocardial localized necrosis (nonfatal MI) and in 1184 patients included in an examination on 5561 British men.

The amount of leptin reduces body weight when using the IF diet. Leptin hyper-action minimizes the danger of atherosclerosis by reducing platelet aggregation and reducing endothelial cell proliferation and migration. Moreover, resistin plays an essential function in the pathogenesis of atherosclerosis. This mechanism is a cytokine gain from adipocytes, and the amounts correlate with resistance to insulin and obesity. It has a proinflammatory action. It also encourages the proinflammatory activity of neutrophils and macrophages and the formation of extracellular deposits in vessels. These occur by inhibiting AMP-activated protein kinase activation, responsible for the inhibition of neutrophil action. Resistin enhances the appearance of chemotactic monocyte one protein (MCP-1) and sICAM-1in vascular endothelial cells. These studies were undertaken by Burnett and his team in which they report on incubated mouse aortic endothelial cells with a recombinant resistin (adipose tissue-specific secretory factor (ADSF).

Research carried out by Bhutani et al. is proof that the Alternating Day Fasting (ADF) diet displays an action in modulating adipokines. Consequently, it has cardio-protective and anti-sclerotic influences. The study involved 16 obese people—12 women and four men. It lasted for ten weeks and involved three phases of nutritive intrusions. The first two weeks were the control phase, the next four weeks involved the ADF diet in which the feeding time was monitored, and the last four weeks were ADF with a self-fed nourishment time by the subject. After eight weeks of using the ADF diet, there was a reduction in leptin amounts associated with reduced body weight and fat content. The quantity of resistin was essentially reduced after using the ADF diet, which is likely associated with a reduction in body weight.

The Influence of Intermittent Fasting on Blood Pressure
Hypertension is a common disease of the modern world. In the United States, this affects 86 million adults. It is a dangerous contributor in cardiovascular disease, stroke, and chronic kidney disease. It is described as the occurance of systolic blood pressure (SBP) at or higher than 140 mmHg, or diastolic blood pressure (DBP) of 90 mmHg or higher. The consumption of an IF diet has a beneficial influence on lowering blood pressure. This fact has been documented in animal reports, and later, the diet's

effectiveness was verified in human subjects. Studies carried out at the University of Buffalo in the United States in male Sprague-Dawley rats demonstrated the beneficial influence of cardiovascular system diet. The animals were exposed to a reduced-calorie diet or an IF. They were fed every day under a circadian rhythm. Telemetry transmitters were fixed to control their heart function. After a few weeks of observation, a reduction in SBP and DBP blood pressure was noted, as well as a decrease in heart rate. The diet benefits have also been verified in individuals in reports organized at the Buchinger Wilhelmi clinic in Germany. The study group comprised of 1422 people were exposed to a one-year follow-up with the IF diet. The Fasting period was about 4–21 days, and daily meals of 200–250 kcal. They examined influence of the IF diet on the cardiovascular system and their findings were consistent with animal studies. The study proved the reduction of SBP and DBP in groups of people who fasted for an extended period.

The pressure drop mechanism may be associated with an enhancement in parasympathetic action due to the brain-gain neurotrophic element (BDNF), enhanced norepinephrine emission through the kidneys, and enhanced sensitivity to natriuretic peptides and insulin. It was discovered that cardiovascular health benefits are not maintained beyond the period of the IF diet. When the regimen was concluded, the pressure values of the participants return to their initial values. The procedure of low blood pressure linked with the parasympathetic system's activation is established on the cholinergic neurons' enhanced cerebrospinal stem activity. Brain-gain neurotrophic element (BDNF) is mainly produced in response to glutamatergic receptors' activation. Still, the IF diet is also somewhat stimulating. The impact of the component on the pulse and circulatory strain has been demonstrated in studies with mice at the George Washington University. Male heterozygous and congenic wild-type mice were examined. In mutual classes, transmitters were implanted to monitor heart rates. Wild-type mice were infused with recombinant individual BDNF into the cerebral ventricles.

In contrast, mice were infused with PBS's mutated solution. After four weeks of observation, it was noted that the heart rate in mice with an intraventricular infusion of the element was essentially lower compared to mice with PBS infusion. Also, the variations were independent of the time of day. Further tests in mice were performed to describe the decrease of the heart rate in the presence of BDNF. Mutual groups were given anti-sympathetic drugs, atenolol, and anti-parasympathetic drugs, atropine. All mice reacted to atenolol, with a decrease in heart rate. However, with atropine, the heart rate was essentially enhanced in wild-type mice compared to the mutant mice. This study proved the influence of the BDNF element on the improved activity of the parasympathetic system. BDNF enhances the synthesis and liberation of acetylcholine by cholinergic neurons. The release of acetylcholine controls the cardiac function through the vagus nerve to the sinoatrial node, reducing the heart rate. Also, the neurotransmitter expands the blood vessels, causing a decrease in blood pressure.

Intermittent fasting Oppose the Deterioration of Cognitive Function caused by Alzheimer's Disease

Alzheimer's disease (AD) is a neurodegenerative disease characterized by a progressive decline in cognitive function linked with neuropathological hallmarks amyloid β-peptide (Aβ) plaques neurofibrillary tangles. Aging is the main risk factor for AD. Limiting nutritional energy intake can slow the aging processes in the brain. It was hypothesized that two diverse energy limited regimens, 40% calorie impediment (CL) and intermittent fasting (IF), could prevent the subjective decrease in the triple-transgenic utilization model of AD (3xTgAD mice). Classes of 3xTgAD mice were kept going on an ad libitum control diet, or CL or IF diets, beginning at three months of age. Half of the mice in each diet group were exposed to behavioral testing at ten months of age and the other half at 17 months. At ten months, 3xTgAD mice on the control diet displayed decreased exploratory activity when compared to non-transgenic mice and 3xTgAD mice on CL, and IF abstains from food.

Overall, there were no prominent differences in the water maze performance among genotypes or diets in 10-month-old mice. In 17-month-old 3xTgAD mice, the CL and IF groups exhibited significant levels of exploratory behavior. They both performed better in the goal latency and probe trials of the swim task analyzed the 3xTgAD mice on the control diet. 3xTgAD mice in the CL group showed lower levels of Aβ1–40, Aβ1–42, and phospho-tau in the hippocampus compared to the control diet group. In contrast, Aβ and phospho-tau levels were not diminished in 3xTgAD mice in the IF group. In this manner, IF may protect neurons against unfriendly impacts of Aβ and tau pathologies on synaptic capacity. It was concluded that CL and IF nutritional regimens could ameliorate age-related cognitive function deficits by procedures that may or may not be related to Aβ and tau pathologies. Alzheimer's disease (AD) is described by the dynamic weakness of memory joined by mental agitation. The behavioral abnormalities in AD result from neurons' dysfunction and death in brain regions involved in cognition and mood, such as the hippocampus, entorhinal cortex, basal forebrain, and frontal and parietal lobes.

In AD these brain regions suffer a degeneration of synapses and neurons linked with abnormal deposition of extracellular deposits of amyloid β-peptide (Aβ), a 40–42 amino acid proteolytic cleavage product the amyloid precursor protein (APP). Aβ may cauterize synaptic dysfunction and degeneration of neurons by inducing membrane-linked oxidative stress, resulting in disruption of cellular ion homeostasis. Transgenic mouse models (utilization) that express a familial AD (FAD) APP change alone or mixed with a FAD presenilin-1 transformation show dynamic Aβ testimony and variable degrees of synaptic disconnection and intellectual interference relying on the specific model. The animal reports suggest that CL and IF may benefit the brain by reducing oxidative stress levels and enhancing cellular stress. Data from individual populations and animal models indicate that reduced food intake may also protect against AD. For example, a prospective epidemiological report of a large cohort in New York City showed that individuals with a low-calorie intake have a reduced danger of developing AD. Other reports indicated that obesity at midlife increases the threat of AD.

Moreover, diseases caused by excessive calorie intake (diabetes and cardiovascular disease) are linked to increase rates of AD. Though CL and IF diets' influences on the development of cognitive dysfunction in AD are unknown, it is established that long-term CL and IF could improve age-related behavioral impairments based on current knowledge.

Chapter 14. A Typical Setup To Maximize Your Results

Okay, now let us discuss the basics of how to lose weight. Generally, you have to eat less than you usually do. That's it. But what is less? You'll need to find your baseline maintenance amount of food - the amount of food that you eat that maintains your current weight. Some people call this your "BMR" (basal metabolic rate); it's the number of calories your body uses if you were to just lie in bed all day. Since you aren't lying in bed all day, you add extra calories to the BMR to account for your usual daily activity. There are mathematical formulas you can use to get a rough number, though these aren't 100% accurate.

What matters is that you eat relatively less than you usually do. Now, I'm not going to ask you to do the math, so go ahead and use Google and search "BMR Calculator" and pick one. Punch in the numbers and get your BMR. My BMR is roughly 1900 calories. If I eat around that number, I'll stay the same weight. To lose weight, I have to eat less than that. How much less? That's up to you, but I recommend not going any lower than ten times your goal weight. Suppose your goal weight is 135; set your calories at no less than 1350. Eating ten times your goal weight will have you losing 1-2 pounds per week. If you eat less than that, you'll be causing yourself unnecessary stress, and eventually, you may have a binge. You don't want that. You want this to be the last time you are dieting. Okay, so now you have your "caloric deficit." That is the difference between your BMR and your diet limit.

What should you eat? Well, you should eat whatever you like to eat, within reason. Still, I recommend favoring protein and veggies, and this will help keep you feel pleasantly satisfied. That's what is great about this way of eating, if you are a vegetarian, continue being vegetarian, vegan, paleo, whatever you want; it's all about that caloric deficit. How do you know you're eating at your deficit? I recommend using a calorie tracking tool for a few weeks so you know what you're consuming. The best app I have found is MyFitnessPal. Set up a free account and track everything you put in your mouth for 2 to 3 weeks. Try to eat a lot of the same meals. Eventually, you'll be able to estimate calories by comparing them to your everyday foods. For me, I don't have to track at all if I don't want to. My regular one large meal and one small meal keep me at my deficit, and the weight falls off.

The last thing you need to remember has to do with weight loss stalls. You might find that your weight loss stops reducing at its usual rate. If it ever stops for more than two weeks, you've hit a plateau. Don't panic! It means your body has gotten used to the deficit, and your hormones have signaled your body to hang on to the weight. All you need to do is take a 2-week "diet break" by eating at maintenance calories (remember the BMR from above?). Usually, this means eating a slightly larger second meal, or at least that is what works for me. After that, drop your calories again, and you'll more than likely continue shedding weight.

Chapter 15. Concerns As A Woman

This chapter is short and sweet. And that's good news. You may have read elsewhere that only men get to reap the rewards of intermittent fasting. That for some reason, because women get pregnant, intermittent fasting causes all hell to break loose! Now, do you think eating later in the day would cause such a disaster? Fortunately, that couldn't be further from the truth. I've found countless cases of women having similar benefits and results from intermittent fasting as men. The only thing I have to say about this is that you should listen to your body and adapt this way of eating to work for you. After you have made that first 2-week adjustment (that period where you will be hungry because your hormones are adapted to not eating in the morning), you should listen to your body and adjust. Pay attention to your work; are you getting spacey or temperamental with your co-workers? That's a good sign you should eat something. If that means you can't stretch your first meal out beyond 2 pm, so be it. Eat! Is your caloric deficit too small? Increase it! Personalizing your approach is the best advice I can give you when it comes to dieting success. You don't want to be suffering, and, for women, compared to men, this can mean choosing a broader window to eat in. Instead of a 16-hour fast, shorten it to 12-14 hours. If a substantial first meal makes you sleepy, eat two medium-sized meals instead, or don't eat carbs until closer to bedtime. One of the hidden benefits of intermittent fasting is it contributes to an increased intuition about what your body needs. Eating the old way, you barely have time to register that you are hungry. Intermittent fasting has attuned me to my accurate hunger signals, to eat until I'm delightfully satisfied and don't need anymore.

Chapter 16. Strategies That Make It Effortless

Alright, so you want to start doing this fasting thing, but you have some concerns. "Won't I be starving and irritable?" "I don't want to go to jail for workplace violence..."

Fortunately for you, after a week or so, the hunger pangs you usually have in the morning will shift to lunchtime (or later). But to make it easier, here are some strategies you can use to make you an IF master.

Get The Weekly Plan Sheet

I put together a 1-week plan sheet that lists my strategy for eating every day. It will help you get through the first week without having to think about the details. A big time saver! Remember, the first week or two will be the most challenging.

Black Coffee

If you're like me, you drink coffee every morning so that this one will be easy for you. If you can drink it black, this will keep your body in a fasted state. If you put milk or cream in it, your body will start to use that for energy instead of your body fat. Which would you rather have? The other benefit of coffee, and the one more relevant to this chapter, is that it blunts hunger. Try it; if you feel hungry, drink a cup or two of black coffee and see how you feel. I find it elevates my focus, so I become a machine at work. No, not a robot, but a highly effective, clear-minded beast! There are some hidden benefits related to caffeine that increase the amount of fat you burn while fasting, but you can find those with a simple google search. We are past the part with all of the citations. As usual, I like to stick with the more practical and obvious benefits, and those are hunger blunting and increasing productivity. Try it; you'll love it.

Seltzer Water

This one is similar to coffee— if you start to feel a little hungry, a little empty in the belly, try drinking a can of sparkling water. The zero-calorie kind that is flavored is my favorite. I drink this cran-raspberry version from La Croix. The carbonation seems to take up space in your belly and kills the hunger. I also just like to have a nice fizzy drink from time to time. Freshwater is excellent, but sometimes while I'm working, it's refreshing to sip a flavored beverage.

A Piece Of Fruit

Okay, so let's say you have made it to lunchtime fasted, but you'd like to push it a little further. Sometimes I want to try my first meal a bit further into the afternoon, like 3-5 pm, but at this point, you're going to start feeling hungry, and it's time to eat. For me, though, I'm sometimes so focused on work that I'd prefer not to cook. Now is the time to grab a piece of fruit from the fridge. Maybe an apple or a peach. As I mentioned in regards to putting milk in your coffee, this will shift your body out of fasting mode, but that's okay; the point of eating now is, again, to blunt your hunger so that you can have even more calories later. Maybe it's a holiday, and you're planning to let loose at the dinner table tonight. Use these strategies to have a large enough calorie buffer that you can eat all you want and still lose weight! Remember, though, and you aren't trying to starve yourself, and if at any point, you start to feel irritable or begin to notice a decline in your work, eat. Listen to your body. For me, if I sometimes want to push my first meal until after work, I might start feeling a bit anxious towards the end of the day, so the fruit brings me back on point.

Meal Sizing

This last strategy is choosing to split your meals' size and it is more of a personal preference. It would help if you are determining what works best for you.

One Large Meal And One Smaller Meal

The one large and one small meal strategy is what I've been using because it allows me to have a massive meal for my first meal, which honestly keeps me satisfied to the point where I usually don't feel much hunger for the rest of the day. I like it because it has simplified my life so much. I only have to prepare one meal per day, and then my second meal is practically a snack− just a couple of small quesadillas or a few eggs and a piece of toast. And if you wanted to, you could swap your meals so the first one is small and then your dinnertime meal is the big one. Perfect for saving up your calories for a dinner date.

Two Medium-Sized Meals

I've followed this strategy for a very long time, and its most significant benefit is maintenance. If you like the weight you are at and want to maintain, have two medium-sized meals. What's a medium-sized meal? It's the usual amount of food you would eat for lunch or dinner, a standard plate of food. You can even follow this plan to lose weight, too, since you'll be cutting out breakfast and eating less. I tended not to lose weight because, as I mentioned earlier, I like food a little too much. So my medium was a powerful medium.

Three Smaller Meals

Everyone is different, and some people are grazers. Perhaps you like to munch on things here and there. A small salad here, maybe a granola bar, some fancy vegan cookies. Now, I'm not advocating cookies, but I know people that just don't eat big meals. It's too much for them. If they ate as I did, they would be on the floor in pain. The Three-Small-Meals plan is perfect for them. You've shifted your calories to the afternoon. By grazing, as usual, you'll have once again achieved that calorie deficit (eating less) that you need to lose weight. The problem with this style is that you might overgraze. At some point, you need to know exactly how much food you put in your body on a typical day. Grazers tend to eat more carb-centric or sugary things, which your body uses up fast, leaving you hungry again quickly. That's why I suggest trying to eat a larger meal with the right amount of fat to keep you nice and full. If it works for you, though, then do it. Keep an eye on your weight and, if you see progress, you're good to go!

Chapter 17. Tips For Intermittent Fasting

Drinking water and organic juices

Many scientific studies have indicated that intermittent fasting is beneficial and has many advantages that primarily benefit the brain and other organs in our bodies. Intermittent fasting induces many metabolic changes in our bodies. One of the most important is that it drops blood sugar levels to manageable limits and cuts down on fat. The drop in insulin levels encourages the burning of accumulated fat. When the stomach realizes that there is no food coming in, it informs the brain, which signals that all the accumulated fat should be used to provide the body's energy. In such a situation, you should avoid drinks that contain "Lucine," which is an enzyme that helps in the synthesis of protein, which would send the wrong signals to the brain.

The brain would react and then send the wrong signals around your body and prevent the breakdown or synthesis of fat. Preventing the synthesis of protein would result in you not losing weight, which would be one of the main reasons to practice intermittent fasting in the first place.

It is as simple as that. That is why intermittent fasting has become very popular worldwide, and many are practicing it very regularly. It is just one aspect of the many benefits of intermittent fasting. There are many more all happening within your body as the homeostasis of the metabolic system is disturbed when regular food intake is denied.

The body is accustomed to the regular three meals or more a day, and the system works with the excess fats being deposited all over the body, sugar levels allowed to increase without any control, and other common consumption behaviours like the uncontrolled intake of sweetened drinks and different types of food that are generally detrimental to our bodies. If these are stopped during intermittent fasting, it gives a wake-up call to our bodies, and then the body has to use whatever it has stored to keep the energy flowing to ensure that the system works at an optimum level. Just because you did not consume a meal or two in intermittent times, the body is not ready to shut down and let you die; it is programmed to ensure you stay alive.

While intermittent fasting may be useful for the body and mind, there are certain precautions. Anyone who is on a fast should avoid causing undo harm from fasting. As you could consume liquids, it would be wise to know what would be acceptable and what could do you more harm than good or, even worse, to make you seriously ill.

Hence, it would help if you took serious note of what you do consume in liquids when you are in the fasting periods. Of course, you should not partake of any solid form meals because you are on a fast. Still, there would not be any restrictions to consume water and other organic juices during that period, but "what" is the big question to consider in your planning.

There are a wide variety of organic juices that you could consume, but it is prudent to know what they contain before you gulp it down your throat. Water is acceptable as you would need to be well hydrated throughout your fast. There should not be any reason for the body to be wanting in water because water is required to ensure that the blood that circulates the body has fluid. Water is essential because it ensures that all the nutrients are carried around the body; it is adequately supplied to all the organs while also taking away the waste from our bodies. Hence water should be taken in moderate quantities to ensure that the above processes are not hindered, which could have adverse reactions in the body. The next question that would arise is how good are the different organic juices and, just to name a few, apple, orange, carrot, tomatoes, vegetables, and coconut water. The critical aspect here would be the quantity of sugar that they contain, and what that sugar would do inside your body. Sugar intake has to be controlled during intermittent fasting. When you are on an intermittent fast, the body is denied sugar, and to counter this. The body produces more insulin to ensure that the sugar within is managed adequately, which controls the "blood sugar" levels. When blood sugar levels are controlled, insulin is maintained at optimum levels and neither increased nor reduced. It is one crucial aspect that is right for your health when on an intermittent fast. You would disturb this equilibrium between "blood sugar" levels and insulin production when consuming excess quantities of high sugar-based organic juices.

High on the list to be avoided is

1) Apple juice, which has 10 grams of sugar in 100 grams of fluid, hence should be avoided at all costs,

2) Orange juice with 8.9 grams of sugar in 100 grams of juice trails a close second, then comes

3) Carrot juice, which has 3.9 grams of sugar in 100 grams of liquid, next is

4) Tomatoes, which is also high in sugar with 3.6 grams of it in 100 grams of juice,

5) Vegetable juice, which has 2.1 grams of sugar in 100 grams of liquid, would depend on the vegetables you choose. The "new kid in the block," which is taking the world by storm for all the good things it has to offer and becoming very popular indeed, is

6) Coconut water has one of the lowest sugar quantities in 100 grams of water, with only 2.6 grams of it just trailing behind the vegetable juices.

Hence it is imperative that if you are on an intermittent fast and need to derive all the benefits from it, you should be prudent in what you consume during and after the fasting periods.

Chapter 18. Pros of Intermittent Fasting

Just like every coin has two sides, nothing exciting or worthy comes with only one side. With all of its advantages, intermittent fasting has its own set of cons too. Here we will look at both the pros and cons of following intermittent fasting.

Pros of Intermittent Fasting

Flexibility

You are entirely free to set or modify your fasting and feasting hours at your convenience. It is not necessary that if one week you fasted on Monday, Wednesday and Friday you need to fast on the same days next week too. It doesn't matter when you fast, as long as you fast for your designated number of hours.

Free Time

Once you start fasting, you will realize how much time you usually spend thinking about or planning your meals. You will be surprised at the free time you are left with when you do not need to prep, cook, or eat every few hours. This free time can be spent on other, more productive activities. A lot of people find this kind of freedom incredibly liberating.

Reduction of Grocery Bills

Skipping a single meal can help in saving a lot of money. Imagine avoiding spending money on your daily coffee or muffin (let's be honest; you spend money on both!). Going hungry for even one day a week will help reduce your grocery bills by a noticeable amount.

No Complications, No Costly Meal Plans, and No Equations: No need to track every morsel you eat. You do not need to calculate the percentages or ratios of the nutrients you consume. There is no need to purchase expensive ingredients or costly meal plans, or fancy equipment. All you need to do is avoid processed foods, eat according to schedule and only eat healthy foods. That's it! While the pros may make it seem like intermittent fasting has no problems, it does have a few in reality. Let us now look at the cons of intermittent fasting.

Chapter 19. Cons of Intermittent Fasting

Difficulty

People who are used to eating or snacking every few hours may find it extremely difficult to adjust to long hours of fasting. The hunger pangs can get uncomfortable, and in some cases, they can even get extremely painful. In some cases to avoid this pain, people usually give up and give in to their urge for snacking.

Lethargy

While this is just a temporary symptom, lethargy is one of the worst side effects of intermittent fasting. Boredom can also be extremely difficult to manage and might cause a few problems at your workplace. It might be a good idea to inform your immediate boss about your dietary change and the symptoms associated with it.

Not Sustainable

While intermittent fasting is highly effective, some methods are not sustainable for the long term. Imagine going hungry for 24 hours two or more times a week. It seems impractical. Such methods can only be applied for a few months before feeling the urge to revert to a more regular and sustainable pattern of eating.

Hormonal Imbalance (Especially In Women)

Most dietary changes impact the hormonal balance in the body as they indirectly influence the production of hormones. It can be easily countered by easing into the diet instead of jumping into the diet. The former gives your body a chance to adjust in time to the new dietary changes.

As you can see, though the cons can have a difficult impact on your life, they can easily be countered with slight changes in your schedule!

www.ingramcontent.com/pod-product-compliance
Lightning Source LLC
Chambersburg PA
CBHW050730030426
42336CB00012B/1501